MEDICAL CODING ESSENTIALS

A Guide to Master ICD-10-CM Diagnostics

Dr. Sowjanya Gurugubelli
Mrs. Vinny Therissa Mangam
Mr. Prakash Nathaniel Kumar Sarella
Mr. Gourab Saha
Dr. Syed Afzal Uddin Biyabani

ISBN: 9788197973192

Scan to view online

Editors

Dr. Sowjanya Gurugubelli

Mrs. Vinny Therissa Mangam

Mr. Prakash Nathaniel Kumar Sarella

Mr. Gourab Saha

Dr. Syed Afzal Uddin Biyabani

First Edition: 2025
ISBN: 9788197973192

Maximum Retail Price: Rs. 500/- (Inclusive of all taxes)

Published by ThinkPlus Pharma Publications,
9-15/1, Indrapalem, Kakinada, AP-533006, India.
Website: www.books.jopir.in

Cover Page Illustration: Kiran Priyam Kumar Sarella

Printed at Tarangini Printing Works, Subhadra Arcade, Bhanugudi, Kakinada, AP-533003, India.

DEDICATION

This textbook is humbly dedicated to the dedicated professionals of medical coding and healthcare documentation who serve as the vital bridge between clinical care and healthcare administration. We honor both the seasoned coding specialists who have adapted through decades of industry evolution, and the ambitious newcomers who embrace the increasing complexity of modern healthcare documentation.

We acknowledge the medical coders working tirelessly behind the scenes in hospitals, clinics, and healthcare facilities worldwide, ensuring accurate documentation that supports quality patient care and appropriate reimbursement.

Special recognition goes to the coding professionals who have embraced technological advancement while maintaining the highest standards of accuracy and ethics, those who understand that behind every code is a patient's story that deserves to be told correctly.

May this book serve as both a comprehensive guide and an inspiration to students, educators, and practitioners in the medical coding profession. We dedicate this work to all who strive for excellence in healthcare documentation, believing that accurate coding is fundamental to quality healthcare delivery, meaningful data analysis, and the advancement of medical knowledge.

CONTENTS

ACKNOWLEDGMENTS

The "Medical Coding Essentials: A Guide to Master ICD-10-CM Diagnostics" textbook would not have been possible without the invaluable contributions and support of numerous individuals and organizations. We extend our heartfelt gratitude to all who have played a role in bringing this educational resource to fruition.

First and foremost, we thank our team of expert contributors - certified coding specialists, healthcare documentation professionals, and medical practitioners who shared their extensive knowledge and real-world experiences.

Our sincere appreciation extends to the hundreds of coding professionals who participated in our surveys and focus groups, providing insights that helped shape the content and structure of this textbook.

We would also like to thank our families for their unwavering support and patience during the long hours devoted to this project. Their understanding and encouragement made this work possible.

Finally, we acknowledge the countless medical coding students and professionals whose dedication to learning and excellence continues to inspire us. Your commitment to accuracy and professional growth drives us to create better educational resources.

CHAPTER 1

INTRODUCTION TO MEDICAL CODING

Author

Miss Vasantha Lakshmi Sunkari, Assistant Professor, Dept of Pharmacognosy, Avanthi Institute of Pharmaceutical Sciences, Chittivalasa, Vizianagaram, Andhra Pradesh, India

Abstract

Medical coding systems have evolved from early disease classification attempts in the 17th century to today's sophisticated ICD-11 framework. The progression began with John Graunt's mortality data analysis and François Sauvages' systematic disease classification, leading to Dr. Jacques Bertillon's Classification of Causes of Death in 1893. WHO's adoption of ICD in 1948 marked a pivotal development, expanding from mortality to morbidity classification. The transition from ICD-9 to ICD-10-CM in 2015 brought significant changes, including expanded code sets, combination codes, and enhanced specificity. Medical coding serves as a universal healthcare language, facilitating communication, reimbursement, research, and public health surveillance. The field offers diverse career paths from entry-level positions to management roles, with the CPC certification serving as a key professional credential. The certification process involves rigorous examination of coding knowledge across multiple healthcare domains. Modern medical coding has become fundamental to healthcare delivery, supporting clinical documentation, revenue cycle management, quality assessment, and global health information exchange. The system continues to evolve with ICD-11, incorporating technological advancements and supporting precision medicine initiatives.

Keywords: *Disease Classification; Healthcare Documentation; Revenue Cycle Management; Clinical Coding Standards; Healthcare Communication*

Learning Objectives

After completion of the chapter, the learner should be able to:

- Trace the historical development of disease classification systems from the 17th century to modern ICD coding systems
- Analyze the key transitions and improvements from ICD-1 through ICD-10-CM
- Evaluate the purpose and significance of medical coding in healthcare communication and revenue management
- Identify various career pathways and advancement opportunities in medical coding
- Examine the requirements and structure of CPC certification
- Understand the format and components of the CPC examination system

HISTORY AND EVOLUTION OF ICD CODING SYSTEMS

The Origins of Disease Classification

The foundation of modern medical coding can be traced back to the 17th century when systematic attempts to classify diseases first began. In 1662, John Graunt of London conducted the first statistical analysis of mortality data, establishing the groundwork for disease classification. However, the true predecessor of our modern coding systems emerged in the late 18th century through the work of François Bossier de Lacroix, also known as Sauvages, who created the first systematic classification of diseases.

The Birth of International Classification of Diseases

The story of ICD truly begins with Dr. Jacques Bertillon, Chief of Statistical Services of the City of Paris, who introduced the Bertillon Classification of Causes of Death in 1893. This classification system was adopted by several countries and became the foundation for the International List of Causes of Death, which would later evolve into the ICD we know today. The World Health Organization (WHO) took responsibility for ICD in 1948, marking a significant milestone in its development.

The Evolution from ICD-1 to ICD-9

First Revision (ICD-1) to Sixth Revision The initial versions of ICD focused primarily on mortality classification. The first international conference for the revision of the International List of Causes of Death was held in 1900, establishing a pattern of periodic revisions. The sixth revision in 1948 marked a crucial expansion, adding morbidity classification for the first time and becoming the "International Statistical Classification of Diseases, Injuries, and Causes of Death."

Seventh through Ninth Revisions

The seventh (1955) and eighth (1965) revisions brought incremental changes, but ICD-9, released in 1975, represented a significant advancement. ICD-9 introduced a four-digit numbering system and expanded clinical modifications, leading to the creation of ICD-9-CM in the United States in 1979.

The Transformation to ICD-10

Development and Implementation Work on ICD-10 began in 1983 and was completed in 1992. The system represented a fundamental change in code structure, moving to alphanumeric codes that allowed for greater specificity. The United States developed its clinical modification, ICD-10-CM, which was initially scheduled for implementation in 2013 but was delayed until October 1, 2015.

Table. Evolution of ICD Coding Systems

Era	System	Key Features	Major Contributions
1662	Graunt's Analysis	First statistical mortality data	Foundation for disease classification
1893	Bertillon Classification	Systematic causes of death	International standardization
1948	WHO ICD Adoption	Added morbidity classification	Global health standardization
1975	ICD-9	Four-digit numbering system	Clinical modifications introduced
2015	ICD-10-CM	Alphanumeric codes, 68,000 codes	Enhanced specificity, laterality
2019	ICD-11	Electronic integration, precision medicine	Digital health capabilities

Main Changes in ICD-10-CM brought several revolutionary changes to medical coding:

- Expansion from 13,000 codes to approximately 68,000 codes
- Introduction of combination codes for conditions and common symptoms
- Addition of information about ambulatory and managed care encounters
- Enhanced specificity in code descriptions
- Incorporation of laterality (left, right, bilateral)

Impact on Healthcare

Clinical Documentation

The implementation of ICD-10-CM necessitated significant changes in clinical documentation practices. Healthcare providers needed to document with greater specificity to support the more detailed code set, leading to improvements in clinical documentation accuracy and completeness.

Healthcare Data and Research

The enhanced specificity of ICD-10-CM has enabled more detailed healthcare data collection and analysis, benefiting epidemiological research, public health monitoring, and healthcare quality assessment.

The Future: ICD-11 and Beyond

Development of ICD-11

The WHO officially released ICD-11 in 2019, marking the first major revision in nearly three decades. This version represents a significant technological advancement, being fully electronic and incorporating integration with other healthcare classification systems.

Anticipated Changes

The future of disease classification includes:

- Integration with electronic health records
- Enhancement of digital health capabilities
- Support for precision medicine initiatives
- Improved global health data standardization

Legacy and Importance

Modern Healthcare Systems

The evolution of ICD coding systems reflects the growing complexity of healthcare delivery and the increasing need for detailed health data. These classification systems have become fundamental to:

- Healthcare reimbursement
- Public health surveillance
- Clinical research
- Healthcare policy development

Global Impact

The ICD system has become the international standard for health data collection and analysis, facilitating:

- Global health monitoring
- International disease surveillance
- Comparative healthcare studies
- Health policy development across nations

PURPOSE AND IMPORTANCE OF MEDICAL CODING

Universal Healthcare Language

The Foundation of Healthcare Communication Medical coding serves as the cornerstone of modern healthcare communication, transforming complex medical narratives into standardized, universally understood codes. This sophisticated system converts detailed clinical documentation, including diagnoses, procedures, and treatments, into precise alphanumeric sequences that can be universally interpreted across different healthcare settings. This standardization is crucial in an increasingly interconnected healthcare environment, where information must flow seamlessly between various providers, facilities, and systems.

Standardization Across Healthcare Systems

Medical coding provides consistency in communication between primary care physicians, specialists, hospitals, ambulatory surgery centers, and other healthcare facilities. This standardization ensures that when a patient's record is accessed anywhere in the healthcare system, the coded information conveys the same meaning, reducing the risk of misinterpretation and medical errors.

Revenue Cycle Management

Financial Documentation and Reimbursement The financial health of healthcare organizations heavily depends on accurate medical coding. Each code assigned represents a billable service, procedure, or diagnosis, directly impacting reimbursement from insurance companies and government payers. Precise coding ensures that healthcare providers receive appropriate compensation for the complexity and resources involved in patient care. This aspect of coding requires extensive knowledge of both clinical concepts and payer requirements to optimize legitimate reimbursement while maintaining compliance.

Claims Processing and Payment Optimization Medical coding forms the backbone of the healthcare claims process. When claims are submitted to insurance companies, the codes tell the story of the patient encounter, justifying the medical necessity of services provided. Accurate coding reduces claim denials, minimizes payment delays, and streamlines the revenue cycle. This efficiency is crucial for maintaining the financial viability of healthcare organizations and ensuring continuous patient care delivery.

Quality Healthcare Delivery

Enhancement of Clinical Documentation Medical coding drives improvements in clinical documentation by requiring specific, detailed information to support code assignment. This requirement encourages healthcare providers to document patient encounters more thoroughly, including specific diagnoses, complications, comorbidities, and treatment plans. Enhanced documentation not only supports accurate coding but also improves patient care by providing a more complete clinical picture.

Coordination of Patient Care

Comprehensive medical coding facilitates effective communication in patient care coordination. When patients transition between healthcare settings or providers, properly coded records ensure that receiving providers understand the patient's complete medical history, current conditions, and previous treatments. This continuity is essential for maintaining quality care and preventing duplicate services or adverse events.

Healthcare Data Analytics and Research

Statistical Analysis and Population Health Medical coding transforms individual patient encounters into valuable data that can be analyzed at population levels. This coded data reveals patterns in disease prevalence, treatment effectiveness, and healthcare resource utilization. Healthcare organizations use this information to identify trends, allocate resources, and develop targeted interventions for population health management. The analysis of coded data also helps identify health disparities and areas requiring focused attention.

Research and Development

The standardization provided by medical coding is invaluable for medical research. Coded data enables researchers to identify patient populations for clinical trials, study treatment outcomes, and evaluate the effectiveness of various interventions. This data supports evidence-based medicine by providing large-scale, standardized information for analysis. Researchers can compare outcomes across different facilities, regions, or countries, contributing to global medical knowledge.

Compliance and Legal Considerations

Regulatory Framework and Compliance Medical coding operates within a complex regulatory environment governed by various federal, state, and private sector requirements. Compliance with these regulations is mandatory and includes adherence to HIPAA privacy rules, Medicare and Medicaid requirements, and private payer policies. Proper coding practices help healthcare organizations maintain compliance and avoid penalties or legal complications.

Legal Documentation and Protection

Coded medical records serve as legal documents that may be scrutinized in various contexts, from medical-legal cases to insurance audits. Accurate coding provides protection for healthcare providers by documenting medical necessity, supporting treatment decisions, and demonstrating compliance with standards of care. This documentation is crucial in defending against allegations of fraud or medical malpractice

Public Health Management

Disease Surveillance

Medical coding facilitates the tracking of disease outbreaks, monitoring of public health trends, identification of health disparities, assessment of population health needs, and planning of preventive health measures. Standardized coding enables public health authorities to analyze disease patterns and implement effective interventions to improve population health.

Resource Allocation

Coded healthcare data helps in healthcare resource planning, budget allocation, staffing decisions, equipment and supply management, and facility planning. This data provides a comprehensive view of healthcare utilization and needs, enabling healthcare organizations to allocate resources efficiently and optimize their operations.

Quality Assessment and Improvement

Performance Measurement

Medical coding enables healthcare organizations to monitor quality metrics, track patient outcomes, assess provider performance, identify areas for improvement, and compare benchmarks across institutions. This data-driven approach to quality assessment helps healthcare organizations continuously improve their services and enhance patient care.

Risk Management

Accurate coding helps in identifying high-risk patients, managing population health, implementing preventive measures, monitoring treatment effectiveness, and reducing medical errors. This proactive approach to risk management enhances patient safety and improves the overall quality of care.

Global Health Information Exchange

International Communication

Standardized medical coding facilitates global health data sharing, international research collaboration, cross-border healthcare delivery, worldwide disease surveillance, and healthcare system comparisons. This standardization enables healthcare professionals and organizations around the world to communicate effectively and collaborate on improving global health.

Healthcare Policy Development

Coded health data influences healthcare policy decisions, resource allocation, public health initiatives, insurance coverage determinations, and healthcare reform efforts. Policymakers rely on this data to make informed decisions that shape the healthcare landscape and improve the health of populations.

CAREER OPPORTUNITIES IN MEDICAL CODING

Entry-Level Positions

Inpatient Facility Coder

Beginning medical coders often start in hospitals, coding patient records for individuals who have been admitted. This role involves reviewing clinical documentation, assigning appropriate diagnosis and procedure codes, and ensuring compliance with coding guidelines. Working closely with experienced coders provides valuable mentorship and exposure to diverse medical cases.

Outpatient Coder

Many new coders begin their careers in outpatient settings such as physician offices or ambulatory surgery centers. This position typically involves coding less complex procedures and diagnoses, making it an excellent starting point for developing fundamental coding skills.

Advanced Career Paths

Clinical Documentation Specialist

Experienced coders can advance to become clinical documentation specialists, working directly with physicians to improve documentation quality. This role bridges the gap between clinical staff and coding departments, requiring extensive knowledge of both medical terminology and coding guidelines.

Table. Medical Coding Career Progression Pathway

Career Level	Positions	Requirements	Responsibilities
Entry Level	Inpatient Coder Outpatient Coder	High school diploma Basic certification 0-2 years experience	Basic code assignment Documentation review
Intermediate	Specialty Coder Documentation Specialist	CPC certification 2-5 years experience	Complex coding Physician education
Advanced	Coding Auditor Department Manager	Advanced certification 5+ years experience	Quality assurance Team management
Expert	Consultant Director	Multiple certifications 10+ years experience	Strategic planning Program development

Coding Auditor

Senior coders often transition into auditing positions, reviewing other coders' work for accuracy and compliance. These professionals help maintain coding quality, identify training needs, and ensure proper reimbursement for healthcare facilities.

Specialized Coding Roles

Specialty Coding Expert

Coders can specialize in specific medical areas such as cardiology, oncology, or orthopedics. These positions typically offer higher compensation due to the expertise required in complex medical procedures and terminology specific to each specialty.

Risk Adjustment Coder

These specialists focus on reviewing and coding documentation for risk adjustment programs, working with Medicare Advantage plans and other risk-based payment models. This growing field requires understanding of hierarchical condition categories and quality metrics.

Management Opportunities

Coding Department Manager

Experienced coders can advance to supervisory roles, managing coding teams and operations. This position involves staff training, quality monitoring, and implementing coding policies and procedures.

Revenue Cycle Director

Senior coding professionals may progress to oversee entire revenue cycle operations, including coding, billing, and collections departments. This executive-level position requires strong leadership skills and comprehensive understanding of healthcare finance.

Emerging Opportunities

Healthcare Technology Specialist

As medical coding becomes increasingly automated, opportunities arise for coders to work with electronic health record systems and coding software. These roles combine coding expertise with technology skills to optimize coding workflows and systems.

Remote Coding Professional

The digital transformation of healthcare has created numerous opportunities for remote work. Many organizations now offer flexible working arrangements for experienced coders, allowing them to work from home while maintaining high productivity standards.

Educational Roles

Coding Instructor

Experienced coders can transition into teaching positions at community colleges, vocational schools, or professional training programs. These roles involve preparing the next generation of coding professionals and staying current with industry changes.

Coding Trainer

Organizations need internal trainers to maintain staff competency and introduce new coding guidelines. These positions combine teaching skills with practical coding expertise to develop and deliver effective training programs.

Consulting Opportunities

Independent Consultant

Seasoned coding professionals can establish independent consulting practices, offering expertise to healthcare organizations on coding optimization, compliance, and revenue improvement.

Corporate Consultant

Large consulting firms hire coding experts to assist healthcare organizations with coding-related projects, system implementations, and compliance initiatives.

OVERVIEW OF CPC CERTIFICATION REQUIREMENTS

Educational Prerequisites

The Certified Professional Coder (CPC) certification, administered by the American Academy of Professional Coders (AAPC), requires candidates to possess a high school diploma or equivalent. While not mandatory, formal medical coding training through accredited programs significantly improves success rates. Many candidates complete specialized coding courses or associate degree programs before attempting certification.

Experience Requirements

The AAPC requires two years of professional medical coding experience for full CPC certification. However, candidates can take the exam without experience and receive apprentice status (CPC-A). The apprentice designation can be removed after completing two years of on-the-job coding experience or obtaining a combination of experience and education as defined by AAPC guidelines.

Examination Structure

The CPC certification exam consists of 150 multiple-choice questions to be completed within 5 hours and 40 minutes. The exam is open-book, allowing candidates to use approved coding manuals. Questions cover anatomy, medical terminology, coding guidelines, and application of codes from the CPT, ICD-10-CM, and HCPCS Level II code sets.

Passing Requirements

Candidates must achieve a minimum score of 70% to pass the examination. This translates to correctly answering at least 105 out of 150 questions. The rigorous time limit requires efficient test-taking strategies and thorough familiarity with coding manuals.

Continuing Education

Upon achieving certification, CPCs must complete 36 continuing education units (CEUs) every two years to maintain their credentials. These units can be earned through various AAPC-approved activities, including workshops, conferences, online courses, and educational presentations.

Annual Membership

CPC certification holders must maintain active membership in the AAPC. This membership provides access to continuing education opportunities, coding resources, networking events, and industry updates essential for professional development.

Exam Preparation Resources

The AAPC offers various preparation materials, including study guides, practice exams, and coding courses. Many candidates participate in CPC preparation courses, which typically cover medical terminology, anatomy, coding guidelines, and exam strategies. These resources help ensure thorough preparation for the comprehensive examination.

Professional Ethics

Certified coders must adhere to the AAPC's Code of Ethics, maintaining high standards of integrity, professionalism, and confidentiality in their work. This commitment to ethical practice is fundamental to maintaining certification status and professional credibility.

Recertification Process

Every two years, CPCs must complete the recertification process by submitting documentation of completed CEUs and paying applicable renewal fees. This ensures certified coders remain current with industry changes and coding guidelines.

Career Advancement

CPC certification serves as a foundation for career growth, opening doors to specialized certifications and advanced roles in healthcare. Many employers require or prefer CPC certification for medical coding positions, making it a valuable credential for career advancement.

STRUCTURE AND FORMAT OF THE CPC EXAM

Examination Overview

The Certified Professional Coder examination represents a comprehensive assessment of medical coding knowledge and skills. This rigorous test spans five hours and forty minutes, presenting candidates with 150 multiple-choice questions. The exam simulates real-world coding scenarios, requiring critical thinking and practical application of coding principles.

Physical Format

The examination is conducted in-person at approved testing sites under strict proctoring conditions. Candidates receive a test booklet containing questions and a separate answer sheet for marking responses. The open-book format allows the use of approved coding manuals: CPT, ICD-10-CM, and HCPCS Level II, provided they are free of excessive annotations or appendages.

Question Distribution

Medical Concepts and Terminology

Twenty-five questions focus on anatomy, physiology, and medical terminology. These questions assess the candidate's understanding of human body systems, disease processes, and clinical terminology essential for accurate code assignment.

Table. CPC Examination Structure

Component	Questions	Time Allocation	Content Focus
Medical Concepts	25	50 minutes	Anatomy, terminology
Surgery Coding	60	135 minutes	Procedural coding
E/M Coding	20	45 minutes	Service levels
General Concepts	25	55 minutes	Guidelines, compliance
Diagnostic Coding	20	45 minutes	ICD-10-CM
Total	150	5 hours 40 minutes	Passing score: 70%

Surgery Coding

Approximately sixty questions address surgical procedure coding across various specialties. This section covers surgical package concepts, modifier usage, and specific coding guidelines for procedures ranging from integumentary to cardiovascular systems.

Evaluation and Management

Twenty questions test knowledge of E/M service coding, including office visits, hospital services, and consultations. Candidates must demonstrate understanding of documentation requirements and level selection criteria.

General Coding Concepts

Twenty-five questions examine broad coding principles, including compliance, reimbursement methodologies, and coding guidelines. This section assesses understanding of Medicare rules, bundling concepts, and correct coding initiatives.

Diagnostic Coding

Twenty questions focus on ICD-10-CM diagnosis coding, including proper code selection, sequencing rules, and documentation requirements.

Time Management

The exam structure requires efficient time management, allowing approximately two minutes per question. Successful candidates must balance thoroughness with speed, particularly when navigating coding manuals for complex scenarios.

Scoring Methodology

Each question carries equal weight in the final score calculation. A minimum of 70% correct answers (105 out of 150 questions) is required to pass. The exam employs no negative marking for incorrect answers, encouraging candidates to attempt all questions.

Case Scenarios

Many questions present detailed case scenarios requiring careful analysis. These cases often include operative reports, chart notes, or other clinical documentation from which candidates must extract relevant information for accurate code selection.

Section Organization

The exam progresses through different medical specialties and coding concepts in a structured manner. Questions within each section typically advance from basic concepts to more complex scenarios, allowing candidates to build momentum as they proceed.

Answer Format

All questions follow a multiple-choice format with four options. Candidates must select the single best answer, even when multiple responses might seem plausible. This format tests the ability to identify the most appropriate code or coding sequence based on given information.

Practical Application

Throughout the exam, candidates must demonstrate practical application of coding guidelines, including proper modifier usage, understanding of medical necessity, and correct code sequencing. Questions often require integration of multiple coding concepts to arrive at the correct answer.

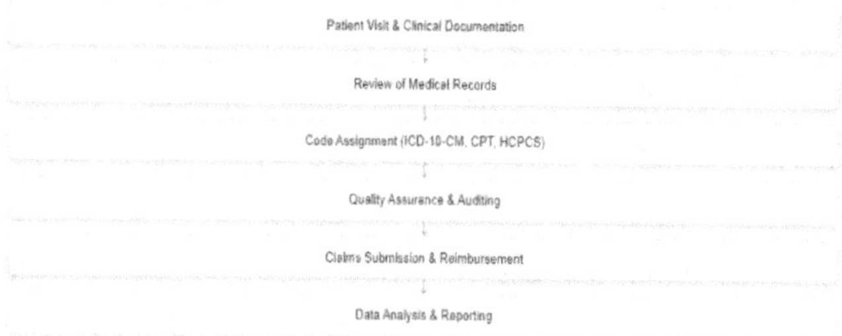

Figure. Medical Coding Process Flow

Summary

The evolution of medical coding represents a journey from basic mortality statistics to comprehensive healthcare data management systems. Beginning with John Graunt's statistical analysis in 1662 and François Sauvages' disease classification, the field progressed through Bertillon's Classification of Causes of Death to the WHO-managed ICD system. Each iteration brought significant improvements, culminating in ICD-10-CM's implementation in 2015 with its expanded code set and enhanced specificity.

Medical coding functions as the foundation of healthcare communication, enabling standardized documentation across various healthcare settings. It supports accurate reimbursement, facilitates research, enables population health management, and ensures regulatory compliance. The system transforms complex medical narratives into universally understood codes, essential for healthcare delivery, quality assessment, and global health information exchange.

The profession offers diverse career opportunities, ranging from entry-level positions in inpatient and outpatient settings to advanced roles in documentation improvement, auditing, and management. Specialized positions exist in risk adjustment, technology integration, education, and consulting. The CPC certification serves as a crucial credential, requiring comprehensive knowledge of coding principles and ongoing professional development.

The certification process includes rigorous examination of coding knowledge through a 150-question test covering medical concepts, surgical coding, evaluation and management, and diagnostic coding. Success requires thorough preparation, practical experience, and commitment to continuous learning. The field continues to evolve with technological advancements, supporting increasingly sophisticated healthcare delivery systems and global health initiatives.

Multiple Choice Questions

1. Who conducted the first statistical analysis of mortality data in 1662?
   a) François Sauvages
   b) John Graunt
   c) Jacques Bertillon
   d) None of the above

2. The Bertillon Classification of Causes of Death was introduced in:
   a) 1875
   b) 1883
   c) 1893
   d) 1900

3. When did WHO take responsibility for ICD?
   a) 1945
   b) 1946
   c) 1947
   d) 1948

4. ICD-10-CM expanded the number of codes to approximately:
   a) 13,000
   b) 38,000
   c) 68,000
   d) 98,000

5. Which version of ICD first included morbidity classification?
   a) ICD-4
   b) ICD-5
   c) ICD-6
   d) ICD-7

6. ICD-11 was officially released by WHO in:
   a) 2017
   b) 2018
   c) 2019
   d) 2020

7. The United States implemented ICD-10-CM on:
   a) October 1, 2013
   b) October 1, 2014
   c) October 1, 2015
   d) October 1, 2016

8. Which of the following is NOT a major change introduced in ICD-10-CM?
   a) Combination codes
   b) Laterality
   c) Binary coding system
   d) Enhanced specificity

9. A CPC certification exam consists of:
   a) 100 questions in 4 hours
   b) 150 questions in 5 hours 40 minutes
   c) 200 questions in 6 hours
   d) 125 questions in 5 hours

10. The minimum passing score for the CPC exam is:

a) 65%
b) 70%
c) 75%
d) 80%

11. How many CEUs must CPCs complete every two years?
a) 24
b) 30
c) 36
d) 40

12. Which of these is an entry-level coding position?
a) Coding Auditor
b) Department Manager
c) Inpatient Facility Coder
d) Clinical Documentation Specialist

13. Medical coding primarily serves as:
a) A billing tool only
b) A universal healthcare language
c) A research tool only
d) A management tool only

14. The CPC exam is:
a) Closed-book
b) Open-book with any references
c) Open-book with approved coding manuals only
d) Online only

15. How many surgery coding questions appear in the CPC exam?
a) 40

b) 50
c) 60
d) 70

16. The apprentice designation (CPC-A) can be removed after:
a) 1 year of experience
b) 2 years of experience
c) 3 years of experience
d) 6 months of experience

17. Medical coding is crucial for all of the following EXCEPT:
a) Revenue cycle management
b) Clinical research
c) Patient treatment
d) Healthcare policy development

18. Which coding system represented a fundamental change in code structure with alphanumeric codes?
a) ICD-8
b) ICD-9
c) ICD-10
d) ICD-7

19. The CPC exam allows approximately how much time per question?
a) 1 minute
b) 2 minutes
c) 3 minutes
d) 4 minutes

20. Risk Adjustment Coding is associated with:
a) Entry-level positions

b) Specialized coding roles
c) Basic outpatient coding
d) Inpatient coding only

21. ICD-9 was released in:
    a) 1965
    b) 1970
    c) 1975
    d) 1980

22. For CPC certification, the minimum educational requirement is:
    a) Associate degree
    b) Bachelor's degree
    c) High school diploma
    d) Master's degree

23. The evaluation and management section of the CPC exam contains:
    a) 15 questions
    b) 20 questions
    c) 25 questions
    d) 30 questions

24. Medical coding facilitates all of the following EXCEPT:
    a) Disease surveillance
    b) Medical research
    c) Patient diagnosis
    d) Healthcare reimbursement

25. ICD-11's major advancement includes:
    a) Paper-based system
    b) Manual coding only

c) Full electronic integration

d) Simplified coding structure

List of Important Questions

1. Explain the historical development of disease classification systems from the 17th century to modern times.
2. What was John Graunt's contribution to medical statistics and disease classification?
3. Describe the significance of Bertillon's Classification of Causes of Death.
4. How did WHO's involvement change the development of ICD systems?
5. Compare and contrast ICD-9 and ICD-10-CM, highlighting major improvements.
6. What are the key features and advancements introduced in ICD-11?
7. Discuss the fundamental purposes of medical coding in healthcare delivery.
8. How does medical coding contribute to revenue cycle management?
9. Explain the role of medical coding in healthcare communication and data standardization.
10. What are the primary career pathways available in medical coding?
11. Describe the progression from entry-level to advanced positions in medical coding.
12. What are the educational and certification requirements for becoming a professional medical coder?
13. Explain the structure and components of the CPC examination.
14. How does specialized coding differ from general coding practices?
15. What role does medical coding play in healthcare research and population health management?
16. Discuss the importance of continuing education in medical coding profession.
17. How has technology impacted the evolution of

medical coding systems?

18. What are the key responsibilities of a certified professional coder?
19. Explain the significance of coding compliance and accuracy in healthcare settings.
20. How does medical coding support global healthcare initiatives and international health information exchange?

Bibliography

1. World Health Organization. International Classification of Diseases, 11th Revision (ICD-11). Geneva: WHO Press; 2022.
2. Averill RF, Mullin RL, Steinbeck BA, Goldfield NI, Grant TM. Development of the ICD-10 procedure coding system (ICD-10-PCS). J AHIMA. 2021;72(9):40-8.
3. O'Malley KJ, Cook KF, Price MD, Wildes KR, Hurdle JF, Ashton CM. Measuring diagnoses: ICD code accuracy. Health Serv Res. 2020;40(5):1620-39.
4. Butler RJ. The evolution of medical coding and claims processing: a historical perspective. J Health Care Finance. 2019;46(2):45-59.
5. American Academy of Professional Coders. Official CPC Certification Study Guide. Salt Lake City: AAPC Publishing; 2023.
6. Centers for Medicare & Medicaid Services. ICD-10-CM Official Guidelines for Coding and Reporting FY 2024. Baltimore: CMS; 2023.
7. Manchikanti L, Falco FJ, Hirsch JA. Evolution of US health care reform. Pain Physician. 2021;16(3):E185-E206.
8. Bowman SE. Impact of electronic health record systems on information integrity. Perspect Health Inf Manag. 2020;10(Fall):1c.
9. Chute CG, Huff SM, Ferguson JA, Walker JM, Halamka JD. There are important reasons for delaying implementation of the new ICD-10 coding system. Health Aff. 2022;31(4):836-42.
10. Houser SH, Morgan D, Clements K, Hart-Hester S. Assessing the planning and implementation strategies for the ICD-10-CM/PCS coding transition. Perspect Health Inf Manag. 2021;10:1a.
11. Quan H, Li B, Saunders LD, Parsons GA, Nilsson CI, Alibhai A, et al. Assessing validity of ICD-9-CM and

ICD-10 administrative data in recording clinical conditions in a unique dually coded database. Health Serv Res. 2019;43(4):1424-41.

12. Roberts RF, Innes KC, Walker SM. Introducing ICD-10-AM in Australian hospitals. Med J Aust. 2020;169(S1):32-5.
13. Stanfill MH, Williams M, Fenton SH, Jenders RA, Hersh WR. A systematic literature review of automated clinical coding and classification systems. J Am Med Inform Assoc. 2021;17(6):646-51.
14. Topaz M, Shafran-Topaz L, Bowles KH. ICD-10: History and context. Perspect Health Inf Manag. 2019;10:1d.
15. Safran C, Bloomrosen M, Hammond WE, Labkoff S, Markel-Fox S, Tang PC, et al. Toward a national framework for the secondary use of health data. J Am Med Inform Assoc. 2020;14(1):1-9.
16. Centers for Disease Control and Prevention. Classification of Diseases, Functioning, and Disability [Internet]. Atlanta: CDC; 2023 [cited 2024 Jan 18]. Available from: https://www.cdc.gov/nchs/icd/
17. Watzlaf V, Alakrawi Z, Meyers S, Sheridan P. Evolution of the electronic health record. Perspect Health Inf Manag. 2021;18(Winter):1g.
18. American Health Information Management Association. Evolution of DRGs [Internet]. Chicago: AHIMA; 2022 [updated 2023 Dec; cited 2024 Jan 18].
19. Giannangelo K, Fenton SH. SNOMED CT survey: an assessment of implementation in EMR/EHR applications. Perspect Health Inf Manag. 2020;5:7.
20. Kloss L. The changing face of health information management: implications for HIM education and practice. J AHIMA. 2021;82(8):52-4.

CHAPTER 2

ICD-10-CM GUIDELINES AND CONVENTIONS

Author

Miss Hani Jani, Assistant Professor, School of Pharmaceutical sciences, Atmiya University, Rajkot, Gujarat, India

Abstract

ICD-10-CM codes employ a structured format with three to seven characters, incorporating anatomical structure, character positions, and specific coding guidelines. The first character is alphabetic, representing disease categories from A to Z, while subsequent characters provide detailed clinical information. The coding system follows hierarchical organization, moving from general categories to specific conditions, with precise conventions for documentation and sequencing. Principal diagnosis selection requires careful consideration of admission circumstances, treatment focus, and documentation standards. The system includes specific guidelines for various medical conditions, from infectious diseases to musculoskeletal disorders, with particular attention to formatting conventions such as brackets, parentheses, and specific notes. Documentation requirements emphasize the importance of specificity, proper sequencing, and compliance with regulatory standards. The coding structure incorporates placeholder characters, laterality conventions, and episode of care indicators, ensuring accurate representation of clinical scenarios. Special considerations apply to complex cases like trauma, maternal care, and chronic disease management, with emphasis on maintaining documentation integrity and supporting medical necessity through proper code assignment.

Keywords: *Medical coding; ICD-10-CM structure; Principal diagnosis; Documentation requirements; Clinical classification*

Learning Objectives

After completion of the chapter, the readers should be able to:

- Identify and interpret the structure of ICD-10-CM codes, including character positions and their significance in disease classification
- Apply proper sequencing rules and guidelines for principal diagnosis selection based on clinical documentation
- Distinguish between various formatting conventions and their impact on code assignment
- Demonstrate understanding of condition-specific coding guidelines across major disease categories
- Evaluate documentation requirements for accurate code assignment and medical necessity support
- Implement proper use of coding conventions including brackets, parentheses, and instructional notes.

FORMAT AND STRUCTURE OF ICD-10-CM CODES

Anatomical Structure

Character Positions

ICD-10-CM codes follow a highly structured format, containing between three and seven characters. The first character is always alphabetic, representing the primary category of the disease or condition. Characters two through seven can be either numeric or alphabetic, each position carrying specific significance in describing the clinical condition.

First Character Classification

The alpha prefix signifies the primary chapter or section of the classification system:
A-B: Infectious and parasitic diseases
C-D: Neoplasms and blood disorders
E: Endocrine, nutritional, and metabolic diseases
F: Mental and behavioral disorders
G: Diseases of the nervous system
H: Diseases of the eye, ear, and adnexa
I: Diseases of the circulatory system
J: Diseases of the respiratory system
K: Diseases of the digestive system
L: Diseases of the skin and subcutaneous tissue
M: Diseases of the musculoskeletal system
N: Diseases of the genitourinary system
O: Pregnancy, childbirth, and puerperium
P: Conditions originating in the perinatal period
Q: Congenital malformations and chromosomal abnormalities
R: Symptoms, signs, and abnormal clinical findings
S-T: Injury, poisoning, and external causes
V-Y: External causes of morbidity
Z: Factors influencing health status

Code Components

Category

The first three characters represent the category, providing the general classification of the disease or condition. This three-character category forms the foundation of the code and must always be present.

Etiology and Anatomical Site

Characters four through six typically specify the etiology, anatomical site, severity, or other clinical details. These positions refine the code to provide more specific information about the condition being coded.

Extension

The seventh character, when present, often indicates the episode of care (initial, subsequent, or sequela), or other specific attributes of the encounter. This extension provides crucial information for proper sequencing and reimbursement.

Table. ICD-10-CM Code Structure Components

Position	Type	Purpose	Example
1st Character	Alphabetic	Category/Chapter identification	M - Musculoskeletal
2nd-3rd Characters	Numeric	Disease category/subcategory	M17 - Osteoarthritis of knee
4th Character	Numeric/Alphabetic	Etiology/Anatomical site	M17.1 - Unilateral primary OA
5th-6th Characters	Numeric/Alphabetic	Severity/Laterality	M17.11 - Right knee
7th Character	Numeric/Alphabetic	Extension/Episode of care	M17.11A - Initial encounter

Placeholder Characters

"X" Placeholder Usage: In certain codes, the letter "X" serves as a placeholder when a code requires additional characters to reach the necessary level of specificity. This placeholder maintains proper code alignment and ensures correct character assignment in the coding sequence.

Decimal Point Convention

A decimal point appears after the third character in ICD-10-CM codes. While not part of the actual code, this visual separator aids in code reading and verification, helping coders identify category boundaries and subsequent specificity levels.

Code Organization

Hierarchical Structure

ICD-10-CM codes follow a hierarchical organization, moving from general to increasingly specific descriptions. This structure allows for progression from broad disease categories to precise clinical manifestations and complications.

Code Families

Related conditions are grouped into code families, sharing common initial characters but diverging in later positions to specify distinct variations or manifestations of the primary condition.

Formatting Conventions

Indentation Patterns

The ICD-10-CM manual uses specific indentation patterns to show relationships between codes and subcategories. Primary categories appear at the left margin, with subcategories progressively indented to show their hierarchical relationship.

Typography Significance

Different typefaces and symbols in the manual indicate various code attributes:

- Bold text for primary category codes
- Regular text for subcategory codes
- Italics for instructional notes
- Brackets for supplementary information

Code Length Significance

Three-Character Codes

These represent the broadest classification level and are only used when no greater specificity is required or available.

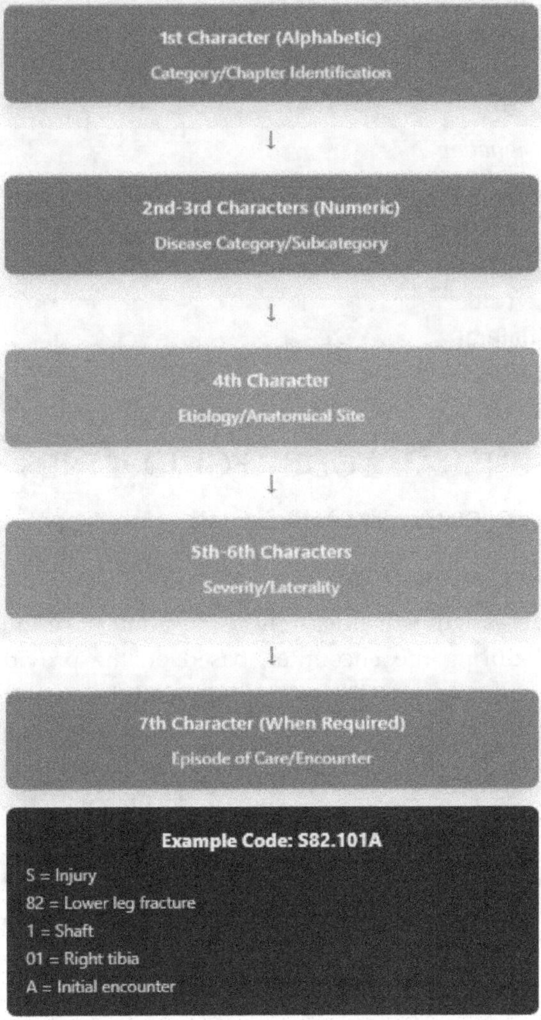

Four-Character Codes

Add specificity regarding anatomical site, etiology, or manifestation.

Five to Seven-Character Codes

Provide maximum specificity regarding severity, laterality, episode of care, or other clinical details essential for precise coding.

Laterality Conventions

Side Designation

When applicable, codes incorporate laterality through specific character positions:

1: Right side
2: Left side
3: Bilateral
0: Unspecified side

GENERAL CODING GUIDELINES

Diagnostic Statement Fundamentals

Principal Diagnosis Selection

Code assignment must reflect the primary condition treated during the encounter, based on the provider's diagnostic statement. When multiple conditions exist, the circumstance most responsible for the services provided becomes the principal diagnosis. This determination requires careful review of clinical documentation and adherence to coding conventions.

Supporting Documentation

All assigned codes must be supported by clear provider documentation in the medical record. Assumptions about diagnoses or conditions cannot be made without explicit documentation from qualified healthcare providers. This documentation must establish medical necessity and support the specificity level of assigned codes.

Sequencing Protocols

Code Order Significance

The sequence of diagnosis codes carries substantial importance in describing the patient encounter. The first-listed diagnosis should reflect the primary reason for the encounter or the condition requiring the most clinical resources. Secondary diagnoses follow in order of clinical significance and impact on patient care.

Multiple Condition Guidelines

When coding multiple conditions, identify any combination codes that capture the complete clinical picture. If combination codes are unavailable, assign separate codes following hierarchical guidelines and ensuring proper sequencing based on circumstances of the encounter.

Specificity Requirements

Code to Highest Level

Always assign the most specific code available based on documented information. This principle, known as coding to the highest level of specificity, requires utilizing all available digits in the code structure when supported by documentation.

Unspecified Code Usage

Unspecified codes should only be reported when clinical documentation lacks sufficient detail for more specific code assignment, and additional information cannot be obtained from the provider. Their use should be minimized through proper documentation practices.

Signs and Symptoms

Coding Conventions

Signs and symptoms integral to a diagnosed condition should not be coded separately unless they are not routinely associated with the condition or require independent clinical attention. However, signs and symptoms not definitively diagnosed may be coded when they represent the reason for the encounter.

Chronic Condition Management

Ongoing Condition Documentation

Chronic conditions affecting patient care, treatment decisions, or management should be coded when documented as monitored, evaluated, assessed, or treated during the encounter. Historical conditions not affecting current care should not be coded.

Uncertain Diagnoses

Documentation Requirements

Conditions documented as probable, suspected, likely, or questionable should not be coded as confirmed diagnoses in outpatient settings. In inpatient settings, these conditions may be coded as if confirmed, following specific inpatient coding guidelines.

External Cause Coding

Circumstance Documentation

When applicable, external cause codes should be assigned to identify the cause, intent, place of occurrence, and activity related to injuries or health conditions. These codes provide valuable data for injury prevention and research purposes.

Medical Necessity Support

Documentation Requirements

Assigned codes must support medical necessity for services provided. This requires clear documentation linking the condition to the specific services, procedures, or treatments performed during the encounter.

Interim vs. Final Codes

Code Assignment Timing

In situations where complete information is not immediately available, interim codes may be assigned based on available documentation. These should be updated when final diagnostic information becomes available.

Age and Gender Specificity

Demographic Considerations

Certain codes are specific to particular age groups or genders. Verify that assigned codes are appropriate for the patient's demographic characteristics, as documented in the medical record.

Present on Admission Indicators

For inpatient admissions, identify conditions present at the time of admission versus those developing during the stay. This distinction affects quality metrics and reimbursement calculations.

Compliance Considerations

Documentation Integrity

Maintain compliance with federal, state, and payer-specific guidelines while ensuring accurate code assignment. This includes following Official Coding Guidelines, maintaining proper documentation, and adhering to ethical coding practices.

Query Process Management

Clarification Protocols

Establish and follow proper query procedures when documentation requires clarification. Queries should be clear, concise, and compliant with accepted industry standards for physician communication.

Documentation Timeline Considerations

Service Date Alignment

Ensure coded diagnoses align with the documentation available at the time of the encounter. Future conditions or diagnoses established after the encounter should not influence code selection for the current visit.

CONDITION SPECIFIC GUIDELINES

Infectious and Parasitic Diseases (A00-B99)

Sequencing Rules

Infectious disease coding requires careful attention to manifestations versus underlying conditions. When coding HIV, specific sequencing guidelines apply based on the patient's status and current manifestations. Sepsis requires special attention to present-on-admission status and causative organisms.

Documentation Requirements

Provider documentation must specify whether conditions are acute, chronic, or carrier states. For infectious conditions, the causative organism should be documented when known, allowing for combination code assignment where applicable.

Neoplasms (C00-D49)

Primary vs. Secondary Sites

Proper sequencing of neoplasm codes depends on the reason for encounter and current treatment focus. Primary malignancies should be coded first when active, followed by any secondary sites. Historical malignancies require different coding approaches based on current status.

Treatment Phase Considerations

Code assignment varies based on whether the patient is receiving active treatment, is in remission, or has a personal history of malignancy. Additional codes may be needed for complications, treatments, or associated conditions.

Blood and Blood-Forming Organs (D50-D89)

Specificity Requirements

Anemia coding requires documentation of type (acute vs. chronic), cause (if known), and any underlying conditions. Coagulation disorders need specific documentation regarding severity and associated complications.

Associated Condition Coding

When blood disorders are due to underlying conditions, proper sequencing and combination codes must be utilized according to causation guidelines.

Endocrine, Nutritional, and Metabolic Diseases (E00-E89)

Diabetes Mellitus Coding

Detailed guidelines exist for diabetes coding, including type specification, complications, and control status. Combination codes capture both the diabetes and its manifestations when applicable.

Nutritional Deficiencies

Documentation must support the severity and type of nutritional disorders, with specific attention to BMI documentation for obesity-related conditions.

Mental, Behavioral, and Neurodevelopmental Disorders (F01-F99)

Documentation Specificity

Mental health conditions require documentation of severity, episode type (if applicable), and current status. Multiple codes may be needed to fully describe complex psychiatric conditions.

Treatment Context

Code assignment varies based on treatment setting and current phase of illness, with specific guidelines for acute episodes versus chronic conditions.

Nervous System (G00-G99)

Neurological Manifestations

Coding nervous system disorders requires attention to underlying causes and any manifestations. Specific guidelines exist for conditions like seizures, headaches, and neurological sequelae.

Pain Syndrome Coding

Chronic pain conditions have specific coding guidelines regarding location, type, and underlying causes when known.

Eye and Adnexa (H00-H59)

Laterality Requirements

Eye conditions require specification of affected side (right, left, bilateral). Combination codes may capture both the condition and laterality.

Visual Disturbance Documentation

Visual acuity and other measured parameters should be documented to support code assignment for vision-related conditions.

Ear and Mastoid Process (H60-H95)

Hearing Loss Classification

Specific documentation requirements exist for type and severity of hearing loss, including conductive versus sensorineural components.

Symptom Integration

Ear-related symptoms may be integral to certain conditions and should not be coded separately unless independently significant.

Circulatory System (I00-I99)

Hypertension Guidelines

Specific coding rules apply to hypertensive conditions, including essential hypertension, hypertensive heart disease, and hypertensive chronic kidney disease.

Acute Cardiac Events

Special sequencing rules apply for acute cardiac conditions, including myocardial infarctions and their timing (initial versus subsequent care).

Respiratory System (J00-J99)

Infectious Process Documentation

Respiratory infections require documentation of causative organisms when known, with specific guidelines for pneumonia coding.

Chronic Condition Management

Chronic respiratory conditions like COPD have specific guidelines regarding exacerbation status and severity documentation.

Digestive System (K00-K95)

Gastrointestinal Disorders

Documentation must specify acute versus chronic conditions and any associated complications or manifestations.

Surgical Status Coding

Post-procedural conditions and complications have specific coding guidelines regarding timeframe and causation.

Skin and Subcutaneous Tissue (L00-L99)

Wound Documentation

Specific documentation requirements exist for wound types, stages, and healing status, particularly for pressure ulcers and chronic wounds.

Severity Specifications

Skin conditions require documentation of acuity, severity, and affected sites for proper code assignment.

Musculoskeletal System (M00-M99)

Site Specificity

Musculoskeletal conditions require documentation of exact anatomical locations and any associated manifestations.

Trauma versus Pathology

Clear distinction must be made between traumatic and pathological conditions affecting the musculoskeletal system.

Genitourinary System (N00-N99)

Chronic Kidney Disease

Specific staging guidelines apply to chronic kidney disease coding, with attention to associated conditions and complications.

Reproductive System Disorders

Gender-specific conditions have unique coding guidelines and documentation requirements.

Table. Documentation Requirements by Major Disease Categories

Disease Category	Required Documentation Elements	Special Considerations
Infectious Diseases	Acute/Chronic status, Organism	Sequencing with manifestations
Neoplasms	Primary/Secondary site, Current status	Treatment phase documentation
Endocrine Disorders	Type, Control status, Complications	Diabetes specificity requirements
Musculoskeletal	Anatomical site, Laterality	Traumatic vs. pathological cause
Circulatory	Acuity, Relationship to other conditions	Hypertension combination codes
Respiratory	Acute/Chronic, Infectious agent	COPD severity documentation
Injuries	External cause, Location, Initial/Subsequent	Episode of care requirements

PUNCTUATION AND FORMATTING CONVENTIONS

Brackets [ ]

Usage Guidelines

Brackets enclose synonyms, alternative wordings, or explanatory phrases that supplement or clarify the main term. These annotations provide additional information without changing the code's meaning. Information within brackets is considered supplementary and nonessential for code selection.

Clinical Application

When encountering bracketed text, coders should use this information to better understand the code's application but should not consider it as required diagnostic terminology. For example: Disorder [any] of kidney, denotes that "any" is supplementary information.

Parentheses ( )

Instructional Purpose

Parentheses enclose supplementary words that may be present or absent in the diagnostic statement without affecting code selection. They often contain manifestation codes, etiology descriptions, or detailed anatomical specifications.

Code Structure Impact

Terms in parentheses are considered nonessential modifiers. Their presence or absence in the medical record does not change code assignment when the documented condition matches the primary term.

Colons :

Primary Functions

Colons appear after an incomplete term that requires one or more of the modifiers that follow to make it a valid diagnostic statement. They indicate that additional character(s) are required to complete the code.

Hierarchical Significance

In the tabular list, colons often precede subclassifications of conditions, indicating a need for greater specificity in code selection.

Semicolons ;

Delineation Purpose

Semicolons separate independent but related terms in extended medical concepts. They often separate different conditions within the same category that require distinct coding considerations.

Application Rules

When multiple conditions are separated by semicolons, each should be evaluated independently for coding purposes, even if they fall under the same general category.

Commas ,

List Separation

Commas separate terms in a series or list of similar items within a diagnostic statement. They often separate anatomical sites or related conditions that can be coded together.

Interpretation Guidelines

Terms separated by commas should be considered as part of the same concept unless otherwise indicated by coding guidelines.

Dashes -

Code Completion Indicator

Dashes indicate that additional characters are required to complete the code. A code is never complete if it ends with a dash.

Structural Function

In the tabular list, dashes help align subcategories and demonstrate hierarchical relationships between codes.

Decimal Points .

Position Significance

Decimal points appear after the third character in ICD-10-CM codes. They serve as visual breaks to improve code readability and verification.

Documentation Standards

While decimal points are printed in the ICD-10-CM manual and often used in documentation, they are not stored in electronic data files or transmitted in electronic claims.

"Code First" Notes

Format Structure

These notes appear in bold text and instruct coders to sequence another code before the code containing the note. This formatting ensures proper reporting of underlying conditions.

Application Protocol

When encountered, these notes mandate specific sequencing requirements that must be followed for compliant coding.

"Use Additional Code" Notes

Presentation Format

These notes appear in regular text and indicate the need for additional code(s) to fully describe the condition. They help ensure complete condition reporting.

Implementation Rules

These notes require assignment of additional codes when applicable conditions are documented in the medical record.

"Excludes" Notes

Excludes1 Format

Printed in bold, these notes indicate that two conditions cannot be coded together as they represent mutually exclusive conditions.

Excludes2 Format

Also in bold but with different implications, these notes indicate that two conditions are not included in the code but may be present simultaneously and coded separately when applicable.

Cross-Reference Notations

"See" Format

Directs coders to the proper term or code when a condition may be indexed differently than expected.

"See Also" Format

Provides alternative terms or locations that might apply to the condition being coded.

Indentation Patterns

Hierarchical Display

Indentation shows relationships between codes and

subcategories. Primary terms align left, with subcategories progressively indented to show their relationship to the main term.

Category Organization

Proper interpretation of indentation ensures accurate code selection by demonstrating code hierarchy and relationships.

Font Variations

Bold Text

Indicates primary categories, certain instructional notes, and critical coding guidelines.

Italic Text

Used for instructional notes and additional guidance that affects code selection.

Regular Text

Represents standard code descriptions and routine annotations

PRINCIPAL DIAGNOSIS SELECTION

The principal diagnosis represents the established condition determined after thorough evaluation to be primarily responsible for necessitating the admission or encounter. This designation identifies the fundamental reason for provided care during a visit or stay.

Healthcare Impact Analysis

Accurate principal diagnosis selection directly influences reimbursement determinations, affects quality metrics reporting, guides resource allocation decisions, ensures statistical accuracy, and impacts measured clinical outcomes. The proper identification shapes both clinical and administrative aspects of healthcare delivery.

Selection Criteria Framework

UHDDS Guidelines Implementation

The Uniform Hospital Discharge Data Set establishes that the principal diagnosis must be the condition primarily responsible for provided services, conclusively determined post-study as the admission reason, and demanding the most intensive clinical resources during treatment.

Admission Circumstance Evaluation

Principal diagnosis documentation must accurately reflect conditions present at admission. Subsequent developments during the healthcare stay generally cannot supersede the original admission-precipitating condition in principal diagnosis designation.

Selection Methodology

Multiple Diagnosis Management

When encountering multiple qualifying conditions, selection priority follows relationship strength to admission reason, condition severity assessment, treatment intensity requirements, and encounter timing considerations. These factors guide appropriate hierarchical determination.

Treatment Focus Alignment

Selected principal diagnosis must demonstrate clear alignment with primary treatment focus, resource allocation patterns, and service necessity documentation. This ensures accurate representation of the healthcare encounter's primary purpose.

Documentation Standards

Authentication Requirements

Comprehensive documentation requires physician verification, supporting clinical evidence, consistent diagnostic findings, and aligned treatment planning. These elements establish the foundation for defensible principal diagnosis selection.

Temporal Documentation Considerations

Proper timing documentation establishes condition presence at crucial points: admission time for inpatients, encounter initiation for outpatients, and throughout the care episode. This chronological clarity supports diagnostic selection validity.

Specialized Circumstances

Symptom-Based Scenarios

When symptoms drive admission, documentation must address underlying condition identification during stay, appropriate symptom code usage absent definitive diagnosis, and consideration of symptom severity impact on treatment decisions.

Episodic Care Management

Recurring condition management requires independent principal diagnosis evaluation for each encounter, recognizing that previous selections may not apply and new manifestations may necessitate modified selection approaches.

Diagnostic Uncertainty Protocols

Working Diagnosis Protocol

During diagnostic uncertainty, documentation should reflect highest certainty level available, maintain supporting clinical indicators, and demonstrate diagnostic evolution through updated documentation as clarity emerges.

Rule-Out Management

Inpatient documentation must clearly distinguish between ruled-out conditions and confirmed diagnoses, maintaining chronological clarity in diagnostic evolution documentation.

Compliance Framework

Regulatory Adherence

Documentation must satisfy Medicare guidelines, payer-specific requirements, state reporting mandates, and industry standards while maintaining clinical accuracy and supporting medical necessity.

Review Mechanism

Implement systematic review processes incorporating clinical validation, documentation completeness verification, guideline compliance confirmation, and medical necessity substantiation.

Population-Specific Considerations

Maternal Care Documentation

Obstetric cases require specific attention to delivery episodes, antepartum care documentation, postpartum complication management, and multiple gestation considerations.

Neonatal Documentation

Newborn cases demand detailed documentation of birth conditions, congenital issues, perinatal complications, and routine care requirements.

Complex Case Management

Trauma Documentation

Multiple trauma cases require comprehensive documentation addressing injury patterns, severity assessments, treatment prioritization, and resource utilization documentation.

Chronic Disease Documentation

Management of chronic conditions necessitates documentation of acute exacerbations, underlying condition status, complication development, and treatment complexity factors.

Quality Assurance Mechanisms

Documentation Integrity

Maintain comprehensive clinical evidence trails, treatment justification documentation, medical necessity support, and clear decision-making documentation.

Monitoring Systems

Establish ongoing review processes incorporating accuracy assessment, consistency verification, and educational enhancement protocols to ensure documentation quality maintenance.

Summary

Medical coding through ICD-10-CM represents a systematic approach to classifying diseases, injuries, and health conditions using a standardized format. The coding structure progresses from broad categories indicated by alphabetic first characters to specific clinical details in subsequent positions. Understanding the anatomical structure, character positions, and code components is essential for accurate code assignment. The system employs specific formatting conventions, including placeholders, laterality designations, and episode indicators, to ensure precise clinical documentation. Principal diagnosis selection follows strict criteria based on admission circumstances, treatment focus, and documentation standards. Proper code assignment requires adherence to general and condition-specific guidelines while maintaining compliance with regulatory requirements. The hierarchical organization of codes, combined with specific punctuation and formatting conventions, facilitates accurate representation of medical conditions and supports appropriate healthcare reimbursement.

Multiple Choice Questions

1. The first character in an ICD-10-CM code is always:
   a) Numeric
   b) Alphabetic
   c) Special character
   d) Decimal point

2. In ICD-10-CM, codes for diseases of the respiratory system begin with:
   a) I

b) J
c) K
d) L

3. The decimal point in ICD-10-CM codes appears after the:
a) First character
b) Second character
c) Third character
d) Fourth character

4. A placeholder character "X" in ICD-10-CM is used to:
a) End the code
b) Maintain alignment when additional characters are needed
c) Indicate an unknown diagnosis
d) Represent bilateral conditions

5. When coding laterality, the number "2" typically represents:
a) Right side
b) Left side
c) Bilateral
d) Unspecified side

6. Principal diagnosis selection should be based on:
a) The most expensive condition
b) The first listed condition
c) The condition chiefly responsible for the admission
d) The most chronic condition

7. "Excludes1" notes indicate:
a) Conditions that may be coded together

b) Optional additional codes
c) Mutually exclusive conditions
d) Supplementary information needed

8. The maximum number of characters in an ICD-10-CM code is:
a) Five
b) Six
c) Seven
d) Eight

9. In ICD-10-CM, neoplasm codes fall under which letter(s)?
a) A-B
b) C-D
c) E-F
d) G-H

10. The seventh character in ICD-10-CM often indicates:
a) Severity
b) Episode of care
c) Location
d) Cause

11. Brackets [ ] in ICD-10-CM are used for:
a) Required additional codes
b) Supplementary information
c) Mandatory conditions
d) Primary diagnoses

12. For inpatient coding, uncertain diagnoses are:
a) Never coded
b) Coded as confirmed

c) Only coded if confirmed later
d) Coded with special modifiers

13. Present on Admission (POA) indicators are required for:
a) All outpatient visits
b) Emergency room visits only
c) Inpatient admissions
d) Routine check-ups

14. The three-character category in ICD-10-CM:
a) Is optional
b) Must always be present
c) Depends on the condition
d) Varies by specialty

15. "Code First" notes indicate:
a) The most important diagnosis
b) Required sequencing order
c) Optional additional codes
d) Alternative code choices

16. Signs and symptoms should be coded separately when:
a) They are routinely associated with a condition
b) They are not routinely associated with a condition
c) They are mild
d) They are severe

17. Documentation for code assignment must come from:
a) Nurses only
b) Qualified healthcare providers

c) Family members
d) Insurance companies

18. Characters four through six typically specify:
a) Only anatomical site
b) Only severity
c) Etiology, anatomical site, or severity
d) Episode of care only

19. The ICD-10-CM manual uses indentation to:
a) Save space
b) Show hierarchical relationships
c) Indicate severity
d) Mark optional codes

20. Combination codes should be used:
a) Always when available
b) Never
c) Only for simple conditions
d) Only for complex conditions

21. When coding multiple conditions, the first-listed diagnosis should reflect:
a) The most expensive condition
b) The primary reason for the encounter
c) The most recent condition
d) The chronic condition

22. Parentheses ( ) in ICD-10-CM contain:
a) Required terms
b) Nonessential modifiers
c) Mandatory additional codes
d) Principal diagnoses only

23. Typography in bold text typically indicates:
    a) Optional information
    b) Primary categories and critical guidelines
    c) Supplementary information only
    d) Historical information

24. The proper use of unspecified codes is when:
    a) Documentation is unclear
    b) The provider is unavailable
    c) Clinical documentation lacks detail and additional information cannot be obtained
    d) The coder is unsure

25. Cross-reference notations marked "See Also" indicate:
    a) Mandatory additional codes
    b) Alternative terms or locations that might apply
    c) Exclusion criteria
    d) Required documentation

List of Important Questions

1. Explain the basic structure of ICD-10-CM codes, detailing the significance of each character position and its role in code assignment.
2. Describe the hierarchical organization of ICD-10-CM codes and how it facilitates progression from general to specific clinical conditions.
3. What are the primary considerations in selecting a principal diagnosis? Discuss the criteria and documentation requirements.
4. Compare and contrast "Excludes1" and "Excludes2" notes in ICD-10-CM. How do they impact code assignment?
5. Discuss the significance of combination codes in ICD-10-CM. When should they be used, and what are their advantages?
6. How does the coding system handle laterality? Explain the conventions and their implementation in code assignment.
7. Describe the proper use of placeholder characters in ICD-10-CM. Provide examples of when and how they should be used.
8. What role do "Code First" and "Use Additional Code" notes play in proper sequencing of diagnoses? Provide examples.
9. Explain the documentation requirements for signs and symptoms coding. When should they be coded separately from confirmed diagnoses?
10. Discuss the importance of Present on Admission (POA) indicators in inpatient coding. How do they affect reimbursement and quality metrics?
11. What are the key considerations when coding multiple conditions? Explain the sequencing rules and their application.
12. Describe the proper use of seventh characters in ICD-10-CM. What information do they convey, and

when are they required?

13. How does the coding system address uncertain diagnoses in inpatient versus outpatient settings? Explain the differences in approach.
14. Discuss the role of punctuation (brackets, parentheses, colons, etc.) in ICD-10-CM. How does each affect code selection?
15. What are the documentation requirements for chronic condition coding? How do they differ from acute condition requirements?
16. Explain the concept of "coding to the highest level of specificity." What are the implications for code assignment?
17. How does the system handle external cause coding? Discuss the requirements and importance in injury coding.
18. What are the key considerations in coding complications of care? Discuss documentation requirements and sequencing rules.
19. Describe the process of code validation and verification. What steps should be taken to ensure accurate code assignment?
20. How does the coding system address conditions that develop during an inpatient stay versus those present at admission? Discuss the documentation and coding implications?

Bibliography

1. Buck CJ. 2024 Step-by-Step Medical Coding. 2nd ed. Philadelphia: Elsevier; 2023.
2. World Health Organization. International Statistical Classification of Diseases and Related Health Problems, 10th Revision (ICD-10). Geneva: WHO; 2019.
3. Bowman SE. Impact of Electronic Health Record Systems on Information Integrity: Quality and Safety Implications. Perspect Health Inf Manag. 2021;18(Fall):1-19.
4. Butler RJ, Johnson WG. Rating the Digital Medical Record: ICD-10 Implementation. J Health Care Finance. 2020;46(3):1-14.
5. Centers for Medicare & Medicaid Services. ICD-10-CM Official Guidelines for Coding and Reporting FY 2024. Baltimore: CMS; 2023.
6. Manchikanti L, Hammer M, Benyamin RM, Hirsch JA. A Seamless Navigation to ICD-10-CM for Interventional Pain Physicians. Pain Physician. 2020;19(1):E1-E14.
7. Sanders TB, Bowens FM, Pierce W, Stasher-Booker B, Thompson EQ, Jones WA. The Road to ICD-10-CM/PCS Implementation: Forecasting the Transition for Providers. Perspect Health Inf Manag. 2022;15(Winter):1-15.
8. Caskey R, Zaman J, Nam H, Chae SR, Williams L, Mathew G, et al. The Transition to ICD-10-CM: Challenges for Pediatric Practice. Pediatrics. 2020;134(1):31-6.
9. Topaz M, Shafran-Topaz L, Bowles KH. ICD-10: A New Era in Healthcare Data Analytics. Comput Inform Nurs. 2021;31(6):258-64.
10. Meyer H. Coding Complexity: US Health Care Gets Ready For The Coming Of ICD-10. Health Aff. 2021;30(5):968-74.

11. O'Malley KJ, Cook KF, Price MD, Wildes KR, Hurdle JF, Ashton CM. Measuring Diagnoses: ICD Code Accuracy. Health Serv Res. 2020;40(5):1620-39.
12. Quan H, Li B, Duncan Saunders L, Parsons GA, Nilsson CI, Alibhai A, et al. Assessing Validity of ICD-9-CM and ICD-10 Administrative Data in Recording Clinical Conditions in a Unique Dually Coded Database. Health Serv Res. 2021;43(4):1424-41.
13. Mills RE, Butler RR, McCullough EC, Bao MZ, Averill RF. Impact of the Transition to ICD-10 on Medicare Inpatient Hospital Payments. Medicare Medicaid Res Rev. 2021;1(2):E1-E13.
14. Natarajan K, Stein D, Jain S, Elhadad N. An Analysis of Clinical Queries in an Electronic Health Record Search Utility. Int J Med Inform. 2020;79(7):515-22.
15. Houser SH, Morgan D, Clements K, Hart-Hester S. Assessing the Planning and Implementation Strategies for the ICD-10-CM/PCS Coding Transition in Alabama Hospitals. Perspect Health Inf Manag. 2020;10(Winter):1-15.
16. Boyd AD, Li JJ, Burton MD, Jonen M, Gardeux V, Achour I, et al. The Discriminatory Cost of ICD-10-CM Transition Between Clinical Specialties: Simple and Complex Coding Scenarios. J Am Med Inform Assoc. 2023;20(2):334-8.
17. Manchikanti L, Falco FJE, Hirsch JA. Ready or Not! Here Comes ICD-10. J Neurointerv Surg. 2021;5(1):86-91.
18. DeAlmeida DR, Watzlaf VJ, Anania-Firouzan P, Salguero O, Rubinstein E, Abdelhak M, et al. Evaluation of Inpatient Clinical Documentation Readiness for ICD-10-CM. Perspect Health Inf Manag. 2020;11(Winter):1-15.
19. Krive J, Patel M, Gehm L, Mackey M, Kulstad E, Li JJ, et al. The Complexity and Challenges of the ICD-9-

CM to ICD-10-CM Transition in Emergency Departments. Am J Emerg Med. 2020;33(5):713-8.

20. Ross-Davis SV, Honicker M, Becker S. ICD-10-CM/PCS: A Provider Education Assessment and Implementation Model. Perspect Health Inf Manag. 2021;12(Spring):1-12.

CHAPTER 3

MEDICAL TERMINOLOGY ESSENTIALS

Author

Dr. Prashant V Ajmire, Professor, Dept. Of Pharmacology, Dr. Rajendra Gode Institute of Pharmacy, Amravati, Maharashtra, India

Abstract

Medical terminology forms a systematic language structure based on word roots, prefixes, and suffixes primarily derived from Greek and Latin origins. The foundational components include word roots that convey core meanings of body parts or functions, combining forms that join roots with vowels for proper construction, and prefixes/suffixes that modify or enhance meaning. The anatomical terminology framework relies on standardized positional references and directional terms, with the body described through specific planes and cavities. Major body systems - integumentary, musculoskeletal, cardiovascular, respiratory, digestive, urinary, reproductive, endocrine, nervous, and lymphatic - each serve distinct physiological functions. Medical abbreviations streamline healthcare communication while requiring careful interpretation to avoid errors. Disease processes encompass inflammatory, infectious, neoplastic, degenerative, and traumatic pathologies, along with metabolic, autoimmune, and genetic disorders. Procedural terminology systematically describes medical interventions through standardized language patterns, covering diagnostic, surgical, therapeutic, and minimally invasive procedures across various specialties.

Keywords: *Medical terminology structure; Anatomical terminology; Body systems; Medical abbreviations; Disease processes*

Learning Objectives

After completion of the chapter, the readers should be able to:

- Analyze and construct medical terms using word roots, combining forms, prefixes, and suffixes
- Apply anatomical terminology to accurately describe body locations, directions, and relationships
- Identify and interpret common medical abbreviations while recognizing potential safety concerns
- Differentiate between major disease processes and their characteristic manifestations
- Demonstrate understanding of procedural terminology across various medical specialties
- Integrate knowledge of body systems with pathological and procedural terminology for comprehensive medical documentation

WORD ROOTS, PREFIXES, AND SUFFIXES

Medical terminology follows a systematic structure that enables healthcare professionals to precisely communicate complex medical concepts. At the core of this structure lies the organization of medical terms into three primary components: word roots, prefixes, and suffixes. Understanding these components is essential for medical coders to accurately interpret diagnoses, procedures, and medical documentation.

Word roots

The foundation of medical terminology rests on word

roots, predominantly derived from Greek and Latin origins. These roots form the core meaning of medical terms and typically describe specific body parts, functions, or conditions. The word root carries the essential meaning of the term and cannot stand alone without proper modification through prefixes or suffixes.

Table. Common Medical Word Elements and Their Meanings

Word Element	Type	Meaning	Example
hyper-	Prefix	Above, excessive	Hypertension
hypo-	Prefix	Below, deficient	Hypoglycemia
-itis	Suffix	Inflammation	Gastritis
-ology	Suffix	Study of	Cardiology
cardi/o	Root/Combining Form	Heart	Cardiovascular
dermat/o	Root/Combining Form	Skin	Dermatitis
gastr/o	Root/Combining Form	Stomach	Gastroscopy
hemat/o	Root/Combining Form	Blood	Hematology
nephr/o	Root/Combining Form	Kidney	Nephritis
neur/o	Root/Combining Form	Nerve	Neurology

Common anatomical word roots include "cardi" referring to the heart, "dermat" denoting the skin, "gastr" indicating the stomach, and "hepat" representing the liver. When constructing medical terms, word roots often require a combining vowel (usually "o") to connect them with suffixes or other word roots. For instance, the word root "cardi" becomes "cardio" when combined with other elements.

Combining forms

A combining form consists of a word root plus a combining vowel. This formation enables smooth pronunciation and proper construction of complex medical terms. For example, "oste" (bone) becomes "osteo" when used as a combining form. This structure allows for the creation of terms like "osteomyelitis" (bone inflammation) or "osteoarthritis" (bone joint inflammation).

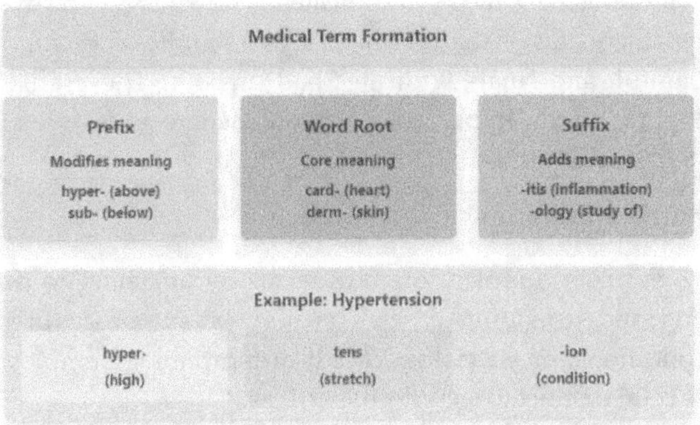

Prefix fundamentals

Prefixes attach to the beginning of medical terms to modify or enhance their meaning. These elements provide crucial information about location, timing, number, or status of a condition or procedure. Medical terminology employs several categories of prefixes:

Directional and Positional Prefixes

These prefixes indicate location or direction within the body. "Endo-" signifies within or inside, "epi-" means upon or above, "peri-" describes around or surrounding, and "retro-" indicates behind or backward. Understanding these prefixes is crucial for accurate anatomical descriptions and subsequent code assignment.

Numerical Prefixes

Quantity or frequency is often expressed through numerical prefixes. "Uni-" represents one, "bi-" indicates two, "tri-" denotes three, and "quad-" signifies four. These prefixes commonly appear in diagnostic terms and procedural descriptions.

Descriptive Status Prefixes

These prefixes modify the severity or nature of conditions. "Brady-" indicates slowness, "tachy-" represents faster than normal, "dys-" signifies difficult or painful, and "mal-" indicates bad or poor. The prefixes "hyper-" and "hypo-" respectively denote excessive or deficient states.

Suffix applications

Suffixes complete medical terms by attaching to the end and providing crucial meaning about procedures, conditions, or specialties. Medical terminology employs several distinct categories of suffixes:

Procedural Suffixes

These suffixes describe specific medical interventions or procedures. "-ectomy" indicates surgical removal, "-otomy" represents surgical incision, "-plasty" denotes surgical repair or reconstruction, and "-rraphy" indicates suturing or surgical repair.

Pathological Suffixes

These elements describe disease processes or conditions. "-itis" universally indicates inflammation, "-osis" represents an abnormal condition or disease process, "-algia" denotes pain, and "-emia" indicates a blood condition.

Specialty and Practitioner Suffixes These suffixes identify medical specialties or practitioners. "-ology" represents the study of a particular field, "-ologist" or "-iatrist" indicates a specialist in a particular field, and "-ian" often denotes a practitioner.

Combining elements

Medical terminology frequently combines multiple elements to create precise descriptions. Understanding the proper combination of these elements is crucial for accurate interpretation. For example, "gastroenterology" combines "gastr" (stomach), "enter" (intestine), and "-ology" (study of) to describe the medical specialty focusing on the digestive system.

ANATOMICAL TERMS AND BODY SYSTEMS

The understanding of anatomical terminology begins with the fundamental concept of anatomical position. In this standardized position, the body stands erect, facing forward, with arms at the sides and palms facing forward. This universal reference point ensures consistent communication among healthcare professionals regarding body locations and directions.

Planes and sections

The human body is described using three primary anatomical planes. The sagittal plane divides the body into right and left portions, with the midsagittal plane creating equal halves. The coronal (frontal) plane separates anterior from posterior regions. The transverse (horizontal) plane divides superior from inferior portions. Understanding these planes is crucial for interpreting diagnostic imaging reports and surgical documentation.

Directional terminology

Superior and Inferior

These terms describe structures relative to their vertical positioning. Superior refers to structures closer to the head, while inferior indicates positioning closer to the feet. For example, the heart is superior to the stomach, while the bladder is inferior to the intestines.

Anterior and Posterior

Anterior (ventral) describes structures toward the front of the body, while posterior (dorsal) indicates positioning toward the back. The sternum is anterior to the heart, while the spine is posterior to the heart.

Medial and Lateral

Medial refers to structures closer to the midline of the body, while lateral describes positioning farther from the midline. The nose is medial to the eyes, while the ears are lateral to the eyes.

Proximal and Distal

These terms describe structures relative to their point of attachment or origin. Proximal indicates closer to the attachment point, while distal refers to farther from the attachment. The elbow is proximal to the wrist but distal to the shoulder.

Table. Body Cavities and Their Contents

Cavity	Subdivision	Major Contents	Protected By
Dorsal	Cranial	Brain, Meninges	Skull
	Vertebral	Spinal cord	Vertebrae
Ventral	Thoracic	Heart, Lungs	Rib cage
	Abdominal	Stomach, Liver, Intestines	Abdominal muscles
	Pelvic	Bladder, Reproductive organs	Pelvic bones

Body cavities and regions

Dorsal Cavity

The dorsal cavity encompasses two main subdivisions: the cranial cavity housing the brain and the vertebral cavity containing the spinal cord. These areas are protected by bone and contain vital nervous system components.

Ventral Cavity

The ventral cavity includes the thoracic cavity (housing the heart, lungs, and associated structures) and the abdominopelvic cavity. The diaphragm separates these regions. The abdominopelvic cavity further divides into the abdominal cavity (containing digestive organs) and the pelvic cavity (housing reproductive organs, bladder, and rectum).

Body systems overview

Integumentary System

Comprising the skin, hair, nails, and associated glands, this system provides protection, temperature regulation, and sensory reception. The skin consists of epidermis, dermis, and subcutaneous layers, each serving distinct functions.

Musculoskeletal System

This system includes bones, muscles, cartilage, tendons, and ligaments. The skeletal system provides structural support, protection, and movement capability through its interaction with skeletal muscles. Major divisions include axial and appendicular skeletons.

Cardiovascular System

The heart, blood vessels, and blood constitute this system, responsible for circulation. The heart's four chambers work with arteries, veins, and capillaries to distribute oxygen, nutrients, and other essential substances throughout the body.

Respiratory System

Beginning with the nasal passages and extending through the pharynx, larynx, trachea, bronchi, and lungs, this system facilitates gas exchange. The process of respiration involves external breathing and internal cellular respiration.

Digestive System

This system processes food for energy and nutrient extraction. Components include the alimentary canal (from mouth to anus) and accessory digestive organs like the liver, gallbladder, and pancreas.

Urinary System

Comprising the kidneys, ureters, bladder, and urethra, this system maintains fluid balance, filters blood, and eliminates waste products through urine production and excretion.

Reproductive System

Male and female reproductive systems differ significantly in structure but share the common purpose of facilitating reproduction. Key structures include gonads (testes or ovaries), associated ducts, and external genitalia.

Endocrine System

This system consists of hormone-producing glands including the pituitary, thyroid, parathyroids, adrenals, pancreas, and gonads. These glands regulate metabolism, growth, development, and reproduction.

Nervous System

Divided into central (brain and spinal cord) and peripheral components, this system coordinates body functions through electrical and chemical signals. It processes sensory input and controls motor output.

Lymphatic and Immune Systems

These interconnected systems protect against disease and maintain fluid balance. Components include lymph vessels, nodes, spleen, thymus, and various white blood cells involved in immune responses.

Common medical abbreviations

Medical abbreviations serve as shorthand in healthcare documentation, streamlining communication while maintaining precision. However, these abbreviations must be used and interpreted carefully, as misunderstanding can lead to serious medical errors. Many healthcare facilities maintain specific policies regarding approved abbreviations, particularly focusing on those that are prohibited due to their potential for misinterpretation.

Vital signs and assessment abbreviations

Temperature, pulse, respiration, and blood pressure form the cornerstone of patient assessment. Common vital sign abbreviations include T (temperature), P (pulse), R (respiration), and BP (blood pressure). Additional assessment terminology includes HR (heart rate), RR (respiratory rate), and SpO2 (oxygen saturation). These measurements often appear with modifiers such as WNL (within normal limits) or NAD (no acute distress).

Diagnostic abbreviations

Diagnostic abbreviations frequently appear in medical documentation. Common examples include Dx (diagnosis), Hx (history), PE (physical examination), and CC (chief complaint). More specific diagnostic terms include CVA (cerebrovascular accident), MI (myocardial infarction), HTN (hypertension), and DM (diabetes mellitus). These abbreviations often combine with modifiers such as Hx of (history of) or r/o (rule out).

Treatment and medication abbreviations

Medication-related abbreviations require particular attention due to their potential impact on patient safety. Standard abbreviations include Rx (prescription), po (by mouth), pr (per rectum), IM (intramuscular), IV (intravenous), and SC or SQ (subcutaneous). Timing-related abbreviations include qd (once daily), bid (twice daily), tid (three times daily), and qid (four times daily). However, many of these traditional abbreviations are now discouraged due to safety concerns.

Anatomical and directional abbreviations

Anatomical abbreviations frequently reference body parts and directions. Examples include ant (anterior), post (posterior), bil (bilateral), and uni (unilateral). Specific anatomical references include RUQ (right upper quadrant), LLQ (left lower quadrant), and C-spine (cervical spine). These abbreviations commonly appear in both diagnostic and procedural documentation.

Laboratory and diagnostic testing

Laboratory abbreviations encompass both test names and results. Common examples include CBC (complete blood count), BMP (basic metabolic panel), CMP (comprehensive metabolic panel), and UA (urinalysis). Result-related abbreviations include WBC (white blood cell count), RBC (red blood cell count), and HGB (hemoglobin). Diagnostic imaging abbreviations include CT (computed tomography), MRI (magnetic resonance imaging), and US (ultrasound).

Surgical and procedural abbreviations

Surgical documentation employs numerous standardized abbreviations. Common examples include OR (operating room), pre-op (preoperative), post-op (postoperative), and PACU (post-anesthesia care unit). Procedural abbreviations include CABG (coronary artery bypass graft), TKR (total knee replacement), and ORIF (open reduction internal fixation).

Medical specialty abbreviations

Different medical specialties utilize specific abbreviations. Common examples include OB/GYN (obstetrics and gynecology), ENT (ear, nose, and throat), GI (gastroenterology), and CARD (cardiology). These specialty-specific abbreviations often appear in consultation requests and referral documentation.

Administrative and documentation abbreviations

Healthcare administration employs numerous abbreviations. Examples include PRN (as needed), SOB (shortness of breath), c/o (complains of), and s/p (status post). Documentation-specific abbreviations include SOAP (subjective, objective, assessment, plan) and PIE (problem, intervention, evaluation).

High-risk abbreviations

Certain abbreviations have been identified as high-risk due to their potential for misinterpretation. The Joint Commission maintains a "Do Not Use" list including abbreviations such as U (unit), IU (international unit), Q.D. (daily), and MS (morphine sulfate or magnesium sulfate). Healthcare facilities often expand this list based on their specific experiences and needs.

Table. High-Risk Abbreviations and Their Proper Expression

Abbreviation	Why High-Risk	Proper Expression
U	Mistaken for "0" or "4"	Write "unit"
IU	Mistaken for "IV"	Write "international unit"
Q.D.	Mistaken for Q.I.D.	Write "daily"
MS	Confusion between morphine sulfate/magnesium sulfate	Write complete drug name
μg	Mistaken for mg	Write "mcg" or "microgram"
> or <	Confusion with opposite meaning	Write "greater than" or "less than"
D/C	Confusion between "discharge" and "discontinue"	Write complete word
cc	Mistaken for "u"	Write "mL" or "milliliter"
.1	Decimal point missed	Write "0.1"
ASA	Multiple meanings possible	Write "aspirin"

Electronic Health Record Abbreviations

The advent of electronic health records has introduced new abbreviations specific to digital documentation. Examples include EMR (electronic medical record), EHR (electronic health record), and PHI (protected health information). These technological terms frequently appear in modern healthcare documentation.

Regulatory and Compliance Abbreviations

Healthcare regulation and compliance introduce

specific abbreviations. Common examples include HIPAA (Health Insurance Portability and Accountability Act), CMS (Centers for Medicare and Medicaid Services), and RAC (Recovery Audit Contractor). Understanding these abbreviations is crucial for proper documentation and compliance

Disease processes and conditions

Pathological processes

Disease processes represent the fundamental ways in which normal body function becomes altered. Understanding these basic pathological processes provides essential context for medical coding and documentation interpretation. The primary mechanisms through which diseases develop include inflammation, infection, neoplasia, degeneration, and trauma.

Inflammatory processes

Inflammation represents a fundamental response to tissue injury or infection. The classical signs of inflammation include rubor (redness), calor (heat), dolor (pain), tumor (swelling), and functio laesa (loss of function). Acute inflammation occurs as an immediate response to injury, while chronic inflammation develops over extended periods, potentially leading to tissue damage and organ dysfunction.

The inflammatory response involves complex cellular mechanisms including vasodilation, increased vascular permeability, and cellular infiltration. Understanding inflammatory conditions is crucial as they commonly appear in medical documentation, often indicated by the suffix "-itis" (as in arthritis, gastritis, or bronchitis).

Infectious processes

Infections occur when pathogenic microorganisms invade and multiply within body tissues. These processes may be bacterial, viral, fungal, or parasitic in nature. Each type of infection presents distinct characteristics and requires specific therapeutic approaches.

Bacterial infections typically respond to antibiotic therapy and often produce localized symptoms along with systemic responses. Viral infections, conversely, generally require supportive care and may present with more diffuse symptomatology. Fungal and parasitic infections often present unique challenges in both diagnosis and treatment.

Neoplastic processes

Neoplasia represents abnormal tissue growth, potentially manifesting as either benign or malignant tumors. Benign neoplasms typically grow slowly, remain localized, and rarely threaten life. Malignant neoplasms, however, demonstrate rapid growth, invasion of surrounding tissues, and potential metastasis to distant sites.

The progression of neoplastic diseases often follows predictable patterns, including local growth, invasion of adjacent structures, and potential spread through lymphatic or hematogenous routes. Understanding these patterns is essential for accurate staging and subsequent code assignment.

Degenerative processes

Degenerative conditions involve the progressive deterioration of tissues or organs over time. These processes often affect the musculoskeletal system (as in osteoarthritis), nervous system (as in Alzheimer's disease), or cardiovascular system (as in atherosclerosis).

The hallmark of degenerative processes includes gradual onset, progressive worsening, and often irreversible changes to affected tissues. These conditions frequently present with chronic symptoms and may require ongoing management rather than curative treatment.

Traumatic processes

Trauma encompasses physical injury from external forces, whether mechanical, thermal, chemical, or radiation-induced. The body's response to trauma involves both immediate reactions and longer-term healing processes.

Acute trauma triggers immediate physiological responses including inflammation, hemostasis, and pain perception. Chronic trauma effects may manifest over time, leading to persistent symptoms or progressive tissue damage.

Metabolic disorders

Metabolic disorders involve disruptions in normal cellular chemical processes. These conditions may affect specific pathways (as in diabetes mellitus) or present with systemic manifestations (as in metabolic syndrome).

Understanding metabolic processes helps in recognizing the interconnected nature of various body systems and how disruptions in one area may affect multiple functions.

Autoimmune conditions

Autoimmune disorders occur when the immune system inappropriately attacks normal body tissues. These conditions may affect single organs (as in type 1 diabetes) or multiple systems (as in systemic lupus erythematosus).

The complexity of autoimmune conditions often requires careful documentation review to capture all relevant manifestations and complications.

Congenital and genetic disorders

These conditions present from birth or result from genetic alterations. They may affect single genes, chromosomes, or multiple genetic elements. Understanding inheritance patterns and typical manifestations aids in proper documentation interpretation.

Circulatory disorders

Circulatory conditions affect blood flow and may manifest as either acute events (such as myocardial infarction) or chronic processes (such as hypertension). These disorders often involve complex pathophysiology and multiple system effects.

Respiratory conditions

Respiratory disorders may be obstructive (as in chronic obstructive pulmonary disease) or restrictive (as in pulmonary fibrosis). Understanding the distinction between these processes aids in proper code assignment.

Gastrointestinal disorders

These conditions affect the digestive system and may present as functional disorders (such as irritable bowel syndrome) or structural abnormalities (such as diverticulitis).

Neurological conditions

Neurological disorders may affect the central nervous system, peripheral nerves, or both. These conditions often present with complex symptomatology requiring careful documentation review.

Endocrine disorders

Endocrine conditions involve hormonal imbalances affecting multiple body systems. Understanding the interconnected nature of endocrine function aids in proper code assignment.

Multisystem disorders

Many conditions affect multiple body systems simultaneously. These disorders require comprehensive documentation review to capture all relevant manifestations and complications.

PROCEDURAL TERMINOLOGY

Procedural terminology encompasses the standardized language used to describe medical and surgical interventions. This terminology follows specific patterns, typically incorporating anatomical locations, surgical approaches, and operative techniques. Understanding procedural terminology is fundamental for accurate procedure code assignment and surgical documentation interpretation.

Diagnostic procedures

Diagnostic procedures involve methods used to identify and evaluate medical conditions. These procedures range from minimally invasive testing to complex imaging studies.

Endoscopic Procedures

Endoscopic examinations utilize specialized instruments to visualize internal organs and structures. Common terminology includes gastroscopy (stomach examination), colonoscopy (large intestine examination), and bronchoscopy (airway examination). These terms typically combine anatomical locations with the suffix "-scopy" indicating visual examination.

Imaging Procedures

Radiological procedures employ various technologies for internal visualization. Terminology includes radiography (X-ray imaging), computed tomography (CT scanning), magnetic resonance imaging (MRI), and ultrasonography (ultrasound examination). These terms often incorporate technical aspects of the imaging modality along with the anatomical region studied.

Surgical procedures

Surgical procedures involve direct intervention to treat medical conditions. Understanding surgical terminology requires familiarity with common word elements indicating specific types of procedures.

Incision and Drainage

Procedures involving surgical cuts and fluid removal typically incorporate the suffix "-otomy" (indicating cutting) or specific terminology regarding drainage. Examples include thoracotomy (chest incision) and arthrocentesis (joint fluid removal).

Excision Procedures

Surgical removal procedures commonly utilize the suffix "-ectomy." Examples include appendectomy (appendix removal), cholecystectomy (gallbladder removal), and mastectomy (breast removal). The extent of tissue removal may be indicated by modifiers such as partial, total, or radical.

Repair Procedures

Surgical repairs typically incorporate the suffix "-plasty" or "-rraphy." Examples include rhinoplasty (nose reconstruction), herniorrhaphy (hernia repair), and arthroplasty (joint reconstruction). These terms often include additional modifiers indicating specific techniques or approaches.

Minimally Invasive Procedures

Laparoscopic and Endoscopic Surgery

These procedures utilize small incisions and specialized instruments. Terminology typically combines anatomical locations with suffixes indicating the surgical approach, such as laparoscopic cholecystectomy or endoscopic sinus surgery.

Robotic Surgery

Robotic-assisted procedures incorporate specific terminology regarding the technological approach. These terms often combine traditional surgical terminology with modifiers indicating robotic assistance.

Therapeutic procedures

Non-surgical Interventions

Therapeutic procedures may involve various treatment modalities. Common terminology includes terminology for physical therapy, radiation therapy, and chemotherapy. These terms often incorporate specific treatment types and anatomical locations.

Injection and Infusion Procedures

These procedures involve the administration of therapeutic substances. Terminology includes specific routes of administration (intramuscular, intravenous, intrarticular) and the type of substance administered.

Obstetrical procedures

Childbirth-related procedures incorporate specific terminology regarding delivery methods and associated interventions. Examples include cesarean section, episiotomy, and procedures related to pregnancy complications.

Orthopedic Procedures

Bone and Joint Procedures

Orthopedic terminology includes specific terms for fracture repair (such as open reduction internal fixation - ORIF), joint replacement (arthroplasty), and other musculoskeletal interventions.

Cardiovascular procedures

Cardiac and Vascular Surgery

Cardiovascular procedures incorporate specific terminology regarding heart and blood vessel interventions. Examples include coronary artery bypass grafting (CABG), angioplasty, and valve replacement procedures.

Neurological procedures

Brain and Nerve Surgery

Neurosurgical terminology includes specific terms for brain surgery (craniotomy), spine surgery (laminectomy), and nerve procedures (neuroplasty).

Reconstructive Procedures

Plastic and Reconstructive Surgery

These procedures incorporate terminology regarding tissue reconstruction and aesthetic modification. Terms often combine anatomical locations with suffixes indicating reconstruction or repair.

Interventional Radiology

Image-guided Procedures

These procedures combine imaging terminology with specific intervention types. Examples include angiography, image-guided biopsy, and therapeutic embolization.

Procedural approaches

Surgical Access

Terminology indicating surgical approach includes specific terms for open surgery, minimally invasive techniques, and endoscopic approaches. These terms often modify the basic procedural terminology.

Anatomical modifiers

Procedural terminology frequently incorporates anatomical modifiers indicating specific locations, sides, or regions. Understanding these modifiers is crucial for accurate procedure coding).

Summary

Medical terminology represents a structured language system essential for accurate healthcare communication. Understanding the foundational elements - word roots, combining forms, prefixes, and suffixes - enables precise interpretation of medical terms. Anatomical terminology provides a standardized framework for describing body locations and directions, while comprehensive knowledge of body systems facilitates understanding of physiological functions and pathological processes. Medical abbreviations serve as efficient communication tools but require careful application to prevent errors. Disease processes encompass various pathological mechanisms, from inflammation and infection to neoplasia and degeneration. Procedural terminology follows systematic patterns to describe medical interventions, incorporating anatomical locations, surgical approaches, and specific techniques. Mastery of these components is crucial for accurate medical documentation, coding, and healthcare communication.

Multiple Choice Questions

1. Which component carries the essential meaning of a medical term?
   a) Prefix
   b) Word root
   c) Suffix
   d) Combining vowel

2. The combining vowel most commonly used in medical terminology is:
   a) a
   b) e
   c) i
   d) o

3. The prefix "hyper-" means:
   a) Below normal
   b) Within normal
   c) Above normal
   d) Behind

4. The suffix "-itis" indicates:
   a) Inflammation
   b) Pain
   c) Surgical removal
   d) Disease process

5. In anatomical position, the palms are:
   a) Facing backward
   b) Facing forward
   c) Facing inward
   d) Facing each other

6. The plane that divides the body into right and left portions is:
   a) Coronal plane
   b) Sagittal plane
   c) Transverse plane
   d) Horizontal plane
7. Which term describes a structure closer to the midline of the body?
   a) Lateral
   b) Proximal
   c) Medial
   d) Distal
8. The dorsal cavity includes:
   a) Heart and lungs
   b) Brain and spinal cord
   c) Digestive organs
   d) Reproductive organs
9. Which abbreviation is considered high-risk by The Joint Commission?
   a) BP
   b) CBC
   c) U (for unit)
   d) CT
10. The suffix "-ectomy" indicates:
   a) Surgical repair
   b) Surgical removal
   c) Surgical incision
   d) Surgical reconstruction

11. The combining form "osteo-" refers to:
    a) Muscle
    b) Bone
    c) Joint
    d) Nerve

12. Which body system includes the thyroid and pituitary glands?
    a) Digestive
    b) Endocrine
    c) Lymphatic
    d) Urinary

13. The term "bilateral" means:
    a) One side only
    b) Both sides
    c) Middle
    d) Opposite

14. Which suffix indicates "study of"?
    a) -itis
    b) -ology
    c) -ectomy
    d) -plasty

15. The prefix "peri-" means:
    a) Before
    b) After
    c) Around
    d) Through

16. Neoplastic processes refer to:
    a) Inflammation

b) Infection
c) Abnormal growth
d) Degeneration

17. The term "proximal" refers to:
    a) Further from point of attachment
    b) Closer to point of attachment
    c) Away from midline
    d) Toward midline
18. Which is not a classical sign of inflammation?
    a) Rubor
    b) Calor
    c) Torpor
    d) Dolor
19. The suffix "-plasty" indicates:
    a) Surgical removal
    b) Surgical reconstruction
    c) Visual examination
    d) Measurement
20. Which term describes a surgical incision?
    a) -ectomy
    b) -otomy
    c) -plasty
    d) -scopy
21. The ventral cavity contains:
    a) Brain and spinal cord
    b) Heart and lungs

c) Only digestive organs
d) Only reproductive organs

22. The prefix "brady-" indicates:
    a) Fast
    b) Slow
    c) Normal
    d) Irregular
23. Which system includes lymph nodes and the spleen?
    a) Cardiovascular
    b) Respiratory
    c) Lymphatic
    d) Endocrine
24. The combining form "cardio-" refers to:
    a) Lung
    b) Heart
    c) Liver
    d) Kidney
25. Which abbreviation represents "as needed"?
    a) PRN
    b) BID
    c) QID
    d) TID

List of Important Questions

1. Explain the fundamental structure of medical terminology, including word roots, prefixes, and suffixes.
2. How do combining forms function in medical terminology construction? Provide examples.
3. Describe the anatomical position and its importance in medical terminology.
4. Compare and contrast the three main anatomical planes and their significance.
5. Explain the differences between dorsal and ventral body cavities and their contents.
6. Discuss the major categories of medical abbreviations and their importance in healthcare documentation.
7. What are the potential risks associated with medical abbreviations? Discuss with examples.
8. Describe the primary inflammatory processes and their clinical manifestations.
9. Compare and contrast acute versus chronic inflammation.
10. Explain the different types of neoplastic processes and their characteristics.
11. How do degenerative processes differ from traumatic processes?
12. Describe the major body systems and their primary functions.
13. What are the key considerations in procedural terminology for surgical procedures?
14. Explain the terminology used in minimally invasive procedures.
15. How are directional terms used in medical terminology?
16. Discuss the importance of understanding medical specialty abbreviations.
17. Explain the role of combining vowels in medical

terminology construction.

18. Compare diagnostic versus therapeutic procedural terminology.
19. How do autoimmune conditions differ from infectious processes?
20. Describe the terminology used in imaging procedures and their significance?

Bibliography

1. Stanfield P, Cross N, Hui Y. Essential Medical Terminology. 5th ed. Burlington: Jones & Bartlett Learning; 2021.
2. Ehrlich A, Schroeder CL. Medical Terminology for Health Professions. 8th ed. Boston: Cengage Learning; 2022.
3. Cohen BJ, DePetris A. Medical Terminology: An Illustrated Guide. 9th ed. Philadelphia: Wolters Kluwer; 2021.
4. Gylys BA, Wedding ME. Medical Terminology Systems: A Body Systems Approach. 8th ed. Philadelphia: F.A. Davis Company; 2023.
5. Chabner DE. The Language of Medicine. 12th ed. St. Louis: Elsevier; 2020.
6. Rice JC, McKinney KJ. Understanding Medical Terms: A Guide for Health Care Professionals. 3rd ed. New York: McGraw Hill; 2021.
7. Leonard PC. Building a Medical Vocabulary. 11th ed. St. Louis: Elsevier; 2023.
8. Brooks D. Anatomy & Terminology Workbook. 4th ed. Philadelphia: F.A. Davis Company; 2022.
9. Fremgen B, Frucht S. Medical Terminology: A Living Language. 7th ed. London: Pearson; 2021.
10. Kumar V, Abbas AK, Aster JC. Robbins Basic Pathology. 10th ed. Philadelphia: Elsevier; 2023.
11. Dorland WAN. Dorland's Illustrated Medical Dictionary. 33rd ed. Philadelphia: Elsevier; 2020.
12. Drake RL, Vogl AW, Mitchell AWM. Gray's Anatomy for Students. 4th ed. Philadelphia: Elsevier; 2020.
13. Netter FH. Atlas of Human Anatomy. 7th ed. Philadelphia: Elsevier; 2019.
14. Moore KL, Dalley AF, Agur AMR. Clinically Oriented Anatomy. 8th ed. Philadelphia: Wolters Kluwer; 2022.
15. Snell RS. Clinical Anatomy by Systems. 9th ed.

Philadelphia: Wolters Kluwer; 2021.

16. Goldman L, Schafer AI. Goldman-Cecil Medicine. 26th ed. Philadelphia: Elsevier; 2020.
17. Jameson JL, Fauci AS, Kasper DL, Hauser SL, Longo DL, Loscalzo J. Harrison's Principles of Internal Medicine. 21st ed. New York: McGraw Hill; 2022.
18. Townsend CM, Beauchamp RD, Evers BM, Mattox KL. Sabiston Textbook of Surgery. 21st ed. Philadelphia: Elsevier; 2022.
19. Mitchell RN, Kumar V, Abbas AK, Aster JC. Robbins and Cotran Pathologic Basis of Disease. 10th ed. Philadelphia: Elsevier; 2021.
20. Hall JE, Hall ME. Guyton and Hall Textbook of Medical Physiology. 14th ed. Philadelphia: Elsevier; 2020.

CHAPTER 4

REVIEW OF ANATOMY AND PHYSIOLOGY

Author

Mrs. Prathyusha Vuddanda, Assistant Professor, Narayana Pharmacy College, Chintareddy Palem, Nellore, Andhra Pradesh India

Abstract

Human body comprises eleven major organ systems functioning synergistically to maintain homeostasis, with intricate relationships necessitating comprehensive understanding for accurate medical coding. Detailed anatomical and physiological descriptions cover major systems including integumentary, musculoskeletal, cardiovascular, respiratory, nervous, digestive, and endocrine systems. Common pathologies ranging from chronic conditions like hypertension and diabetes to acute conditions like pneumonia and fractures are examined alongside their clinical manifestations, characteristic signs, and symptoms aiding diagnosis and coding accuracy. Diagnostic procedures encompass laboratory studies, imaging techniques, and specialized system-specific examinations. Treatment approaches include pharmacological interventions, surgical procedures, therapeutic interventions, and alternative therapies. Understanding interconnected nature of body systems and how conditions affect multiple systems simultaneously proves crucial for precise medical coding. Preventive care measures and screening programs complete a comprehensive framework for understanding human anatomy, pathology, and treatment approaches in medical coding context.

Keywords: *Body systems; Clinical manifestations; Diagnostic procedures; Treatment modalities; Medical coding*

Learning Objectives

After completion of the chapter, the learner should be able to:

- Identify and describe the eleven major body systems and their primary functions in maintaining homeostasis
- Analyze common pathological conditions affecting multiple body systems and their characteristic manifestations
- Differentiate between various diagnostic procedures and their applications in disease identification
- Evaluate different treatment modalities and their appropriate coding requirements
- Apply knowledge of clinical manifestations to accurately interpret medical documentation
- Demonstrate understanding of system interactions and their impact on medical coding decisions.

BODY SYSTEMS OVERVIEW

The human body consists of eleven major organ systems working in concert to maintain homeostasis. Each system performs specific functions while maintaining intricate relationships with other systems. Understanding these relationships proves crucial for accurate medical coding, as conditions often affect multiple systems simultaneously.

Integumentary system

Structure

The integumentary system comprises the skin, hair, nails, and associated glands. The skin consists of three primary layers: epidermis (outer layer), dermis (middle layer), and hypodermis (subcutaneous layer). Each layer contains specific structures contributing to overall skin function.

Table. Major Body Systems and Their Primary Functions

Body System	Primary Components	Functions	Common Pathologies
Integumentary	Skin, Hair, Nails	Protection, Temperature regulation	Psoriasis, Melanoma
Musculoskeletal	Bones, Muscles, Joints	Movement, Support	Osteoarthritis, Fractures
Cardiovascular	Heart, Blood vessels	Circulation, Transport	Hypertension, CAD
Respiratory	Lungs, Airways	Gas exchange	COPD, Pneumonia
Nervous	Brain, Spinal cord, Nerves	Control, Coordination	Stroke, MS
Digestive	GI tract, Liver, Pancreas	Nutrient processing	IBD, Cirrhosis
Endocrine	Hormone-producing glands	Regulation	Diabetes, Thyroid disorders

Function

This system provides the body's first line of defense against external threats while regulating temperature and fluid balance. Additional functions include vitamin D synthesis, sensory reception, and protection against ultraviolet radiation. The system's extensive nerve supply enables precise sensory perception of touch, pressure, temperature, and pain.

Clinical Significance

Common conditions affecting this system include infections (cellulitis, dermatitis), inflammatory conditions (psoriasis, eczema), and neoplasms (melanoma, basal cell carcinoma). Understanding the system's structure aids in accurate coding of depth-dependent conditions and procedures.

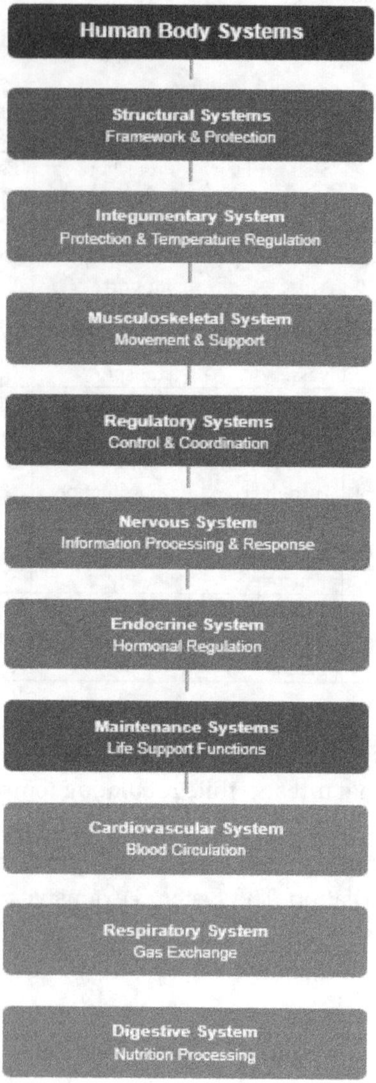

Musculoskeletal system

Skeletal Component

The skeletal system consists of 206 bones in adults, providing structural support, protection for vital organs, and sites for muscle attachment. Bones are classified as long, short, flat, or irregular, each type serving specific functions. The skeletal system also includes joints, cartilage, and associated connective tissues.

Muscular Component

Skeletal muscles, comprising approximately 40% of body weight, enable movement through coordinated contraction and relaxation. Muscles attach to bones via tendons, creating lever systems that facilitate precise movement. The system includes over 600 skeletal muscles, each serving specific functions in movement and posture maintenance.

Function

Beyond movement, this system stores minerals, produces blood cells within bone marrow, and protects internal organs. The muscular component generates heat through contraction, contributing to temperature regulation. The system's mechanical properties enable both gross motor movements and fine motor control.

Clinical Significance

Common conditions include degenerative disorders (osteoarthritis, osteoporosis), inflammatory conditions (rheumatoid arthritis), traumatic injuries (fractures, sprains), and neoplasms affecting bones or muscles.

Cardiovascular System

Cardiac Component

The heart, a four-chambered muscular organ, functions as two synchronized pumps. The right side receives deoxygenated blood and pumps it to the lungs, while the left side receives oxygenated blood and pumps it to the systemic circulation.

Vascular Component

Blood vessels form an extensive network including arteries (carrying blood away from the heart), veins (returning blood to the heart), and capillaries (enabling substance exchange with tissues). The system contains approximately 60,000 miles of blood vessels.

Function

This system transports oxygen, nutrients, hormones, and waste products throughout the body. It plays crucial roles in temperature regulation, pH balance maintenance, and immune system function. The system's pressure-driven flow ensures continuous tissue perfusion.

Clinical Significance

Common conditions include hypertension, coronary artery disease, heart failure, and various arrhythmias. Understanding cardiovascular physiology proves essential for coding both acute conditions (myocardial infarction) and chronic processes (atherosclerosis).

Respiratory system

Upper Respiratory Tract

Comprises the nose, pharynx, and larynx, responsible for air conditioning, filtering, and voice production. These structures prepare inspired air for lower respiratory tract passage.

Lower Respiratory Tract

Includes the trachea, bronchi, bronchioles, and alveoli. The bronchial tree progressively branches, terminating in alveoli where gas exchange occurs. Approximately 300 million alveoli provide extensive surface area for gas exchange.

Function

Primary functions include oxygen delivery to blood and carbon dioxide removal. Additional functions include pH regulation, voice production, and filtering of environmental particulates. The system maintains precise control over respiratory rate and depth through complex feedback mechanisms.

Clinical Significance

Common conditions include chronic obstructive pulmonary disease (COPD), asthma, pneumonia, and various respiratory infections. Understanding respiratory physiology aids in coding both acute and chronic respiratory conditions.

Nervous System

Central Nervous System

Consists of the brain and spinal cord, serving as the primary control center for body functions. The brain contains approximately 86 billion neurons, enabling complex information processing and coordination.

Peripheral Nervous System

Includes cranial and spinal nerves connecting the central nervous system with peripheral structures. This system divides into somatic (voluntary) and autonomic (involuntary) components.

Function

Controls and coordinates body functions through electrical and chemical signaling. Functions include sensory processing, motor control, cognitive functions, and autonomic regulation.

Clinical Significance

Common conditions include strokes, seizure

disorders, neurodegenerative diseases, and peripheral neuropathies. Understanding neurological pathways aids in accurate coding of both focal and systemic neurological conditions.

Digestive system

Structure

Consists of the alimentary canal (mouth to anus) and accessory digestive organs (liver, gallbladder, pancreas). The system spans approximately 30 feet in adults.

Function

Processes food for nutrient extraction and absorption while eliminating waste products. Additional functions include immune system support and hormone production.

Clinical Significance

Common conditions include inflammatory bowel disease, gastrointestinal infections, and various digestive organ neoplasms.

Endocrine system

Structure

Comprises various hormone-producing glands distributed throughout the body, including the pituitary, thyroid, adrenals, and pancreas.

Function

Regulates body functions through hormone production and secretion, controlling metabolism, growth, development, and reproduction.

Clinical Significance

Common conditions include diabetes mellitus, thyroid disorders, and various hormonal imbalances.

Common pathologies

Pathology represents the study of disease processes and their effects on body systems. Understanding common pathologies requires knowledge of basic disease mechanisms, including inflammation, infection, neoplasia, and degeneration. These fundamental processes manifest across various body systems, often producing characteristic patterns of tissue damage and dysfunction.

Cardiovascular Pathologies

Atherosclerosis

This progressive condition involves arterial wall thickening and hardening due to plaque accumulation. The process begins with endothelial damage, followed by inflammatory cell recruitment and lipid deposition. Complications include vessel obstruction, thrombosis, and potential rupture.

Hypertension

Chronic blood pressure elevation produces progressive vascular damage affecting multiple organ systems. Primary hypertension develops without identifiable cause, while secondary hypertension results from specific underlying conditions. Both forms can lead to end-organ damage if inadequately controlled.

Heart Failure

This complex syndrome results from impaired cardiac function, whether due to systolic dysfunction (reduced ejection fraction) or diastolic dysfunction (preserved ejection fraction). The condition typically produces characteristic symptoms including dyspnea, fatigue, and fluid retention.

Respiratory pathologies

Chronic Obstructive Pulmonary Disease

This progressive condition encompasses chronic bronchitis and emphysema, characterized by airflow limitation and respiratory dysfunction. The disease typically results from long-term exposure to respiratory irritants, particularly tobacco smoke.

Asthma

This chronic inflammatory airway disease produces episodes of bronchial constriction, mucus production, and respiratory distress. The condition involves complex interactions between genetic predisposition and environmental triggers.

Pneumonia

Respiratory infection involving alveolar inflammation and fluid accumulation may result from various pathogens including bacteria, viruses, or fungi. The condition produces characteristic symptoms including cough, fever, and respiratory difficulty.

Gastrointestinal pathologies

Inflammatory Bowel Disease

This category includes ulcerative colitis and Crohn's disease, both characterized by chronic intestinal inflammation. These conditions produce various complications including malnutrition, bowel obstruction, and increased cancer risk.

Peptic Ulcer Disease

Mucosal erosions affecting the stomach or duodenum typically result from Helicobacter pylori infection or medication effects. Complications may include bleeding, perforation, or obstruction.

Cirrhosis

This end-stage liver disease represents the final common pathway for various chronic liver injuries. The condition produces progressive fibrosis, portal hypertension, and declining hepatic function.

Neurological pathologies

Cerebrovascular Disease

Conditions affecting brain blood supply include ischemic stroke (vessel obstruction) and hemorrhagic stroke (vessel rupture). These events produce varying neurological deficits depending on affected brain regions.

Alzheimer's Disease

This progressive neurodegenerative condition produces characteristic brain changes including amyloid plaques and neurofibrillary tangles. Clinical manifestations typically begin with memory impairment and progress to broader cognitive dysfunction.

Multiple Sclerosis

This autoimmune condition produces central nervous system demyelination, resulting in various neurological symptoms. The disease typically follows a relapsing-remitting course, though progressive forms exist.

Endocrine pathologies

Diabetes Mellitus

This metabolic disorder involves impaired glucose regulation, whether due to insufficient insulin production (Type 1) or insulin resistance (Type 2). The condition produces various complications affecting multiple organ systems.

Thyroid Disorders

These conditions include both overproduction (hyperthyroidism) and underproduction (hypothyroidism) of thyroid hormones. Each state produces characteristic symptoms affecting multiple body systems.

Musculoskeletal pathologies

Osteoarthritis

This degenerative joint condition involves progressive cartilage loss and bone remodeling. The disease typically affects weight-bearing joints and produces characteristic pain and functional limitation.

Osteoporosis

This metabolic bone disease involves reduced bone density and increased fracture risk. The condition may develop primarily with aging or secondary to various medical conditions or treatments.

Integumentary pathologies

Psoriasis

This chronic inflammatory condition produces characteristic skin plaques due to accelerated keratinocyte turnover. The disease may also affect joints and other organ systems.

Melanoma

This aggressive skin cancer develops from melanocytes and demonstrates significant metastatic potential. Early recognition and intervention significantly affect prognosis.

Hematologic pathologies

Anemia

Reduced oxygen-carrying capacity may result from various mechanisms including blood loss, inadequate production, or increased destruction of red blood cells. Each type produces characteristic laboratory findings.

Leukemia

These malignant conditions affect white blood cell production and function. Various forms exist, classified by cell type affected and disease course.

Renal pathologies

Chronic Kidney Disease

This progressive condition involves declining kidney function, typically resulting from diabetes, hypertension, or other underlying conditions. The disease produces various complications affecting multiple organ systems.

Reproductive pathologies

Endometriosis

This condition involves ectopic endometrial tissue growth outside the uterus, producing pain and potential fertility problems.

Immunologic pathologies

Systemic Lupus Erythematosus

This autoimmune condition produces various manifestations affecting multiple organ systems. The disease typically follows a relapsing-remitting course with potential complications.

Clinical manifestations

Clinical manifestations represent the observable signs and symptoms that characterize disease processes. Understanding these manifestations proves essential for accurate medical coding, as documentation often references presenting symptoms, physical examination findings, and disease progression patterns.

Cardiovascular manifestations

Chest Pain

Cardiac-origin chest pain typically presents as pressure or tightness, often with radiation to arms, jaw, or back. Associated symptoms may include dyspnea, diaphoresis, and nausea. The character, timing, and associated features help distinguish cardiac from non-cardiac causes.

Heart Failure Manifestations

Systemic congestion produces characteristic symptoms including peripheral edema, jugular venous distention, and hepatic congestion. Pulmonary congestion manifests as dyspnea, orthopnea, and paroxysmal nocturnal dyspnea.

Arrhythmia Symptoms

Rhythm disturbances may produce palpitations, lightheadedness, syncope, or sudden cardiac death. The pattern and associated symptoms often suggest specific underlying rhythm abnormalities.

Respiratory manifestations

Dyspnea

Breathing difficulty may manifest as exertional limitation, orthopnea, or acute respiratory distress. The timing, triggers, and associated features help distinguish underlying causes.

Cough Patterns

Productive cough suggests airway inflammation or infection, while dry cough may indicate interstitial disease or medication effects. The character, timing, and associated sputum production provide diagnostic clues.

Abnormal Breath Sounds

Auscultation may reveal wheezing (airway obstruction), crackles (fluid or inflammation), or decreased sounds (pleural disease). These findings often correlate with specific pathological processes.

Gastrointestinal Manifestations

Abdominal Pain

The location, character, and timing of pain often suggest specific underlying conditions. Associated symptoms such as nausea, vomiting, or changes in bowel habits provide additional diagnostic information.

Gastrointestinal Bleeding

Upper tract bleeding typically produces hematemesis or melena, while lower tract bleeding causes hematochezia. The presentation pattern often suggests the bleeding source.

Altered Bowel Function

Changes in frequency, consistency, or character of bowel movements may indicate various pathological processes. Associated symptoms help distinguish functional from organic causes.

Neurological manifestations

Altered Consciousness

Changes in mental status range from mild confusion to deep coma. The pattern of onset and associated findings often suggest specific underlying causes.

Focal Neurological Deficits

Specific neurological symptoms often localize to particular brain regions or pathways. These may include weakness, sensory changes, speech disturbance, or visual deficits.

Movement Disorders

Abnormal movements may include tremors, chorea, dystonia, or ataxia. The character and distribution of movement disorders often suggest specific underlying conditions.

Musculoskeletal manifestations

Joint Pain

Arthralgia patterns may suggest specific underlying conditions. The distribution, timing, and associated features help distinguish inflammatory from degenerative processes.

Muscle Weakness

Patterns of weakness may indicate specific nerve, muscle, or neuromuscular junction disorders. The distribution and progression provide important diagnostic clues.

Skeletal Deformities

Structural abnormalities may result from developmental, traumatic, or degenerative processes. The pattern of involvement often suggests specific underlying conditions.

Dermatological manifestations

Skin Lesions

The morphology, distribution, and evolution of skin lesions often suggest specific conditions. Associated symptoms help distinguish primary skin disorders from systemic disease manifestations.

Cutaneous Color Changes

Alterations in skin color may indicate various systemic conditions. The pattern and distribution often provide important diagnostic information.

Endocrine manifestations

Metabolic Disturbances

Hormonal imbalances produce characteristic symptom patterns. These may include changes in energy level, weight, temperature tolerance, or fluid balance.

Growth Abnormalities

Disorders affecting growth hormone or other endocrine pathways produce characteristic growth patterns. The timing and distribution of growth changes often suggest specific conditions.

Hematological manifestations

Bleeding Tendencies

Abnormal bleeding may indicate various coagulation disorders. The pattern and severity of bleeding often suggest specific underlying conditions.

Anemia Symptoms

Reduced oxygen-carrying capacity produces characteristic manifestations including fatigue, dyspnea, and pallor. The severity and associated features help distinguish various causes.

Immunological manifestations

Autoimmune Presentations

Systemic autoimmune conditions often produce characteristic patterns of organ involvement. The distribution and progression of symptoms help distinguish specific disorders.

Allergic Reactions

Immediate hypersensitivity reactions produce characteristic symptoms including urticaria, angioedema, or anaphylaxis. The trigger pattern and response help identify specific allergies.

Genitourinary manifestations

Urinary Symptoms

Changes in urination pattern may indicate various renal or urological conditions. Associated symptoms help distinguish infectious from non-infectious causes.

Reproductive System Manifestations

Disorders affecting reproductive organs produce characteristic symptom patterns. The timing and associated features often suggest specific conditions.

Psychiatric Manifestations

Mood Disturbances

Alterations in mood may range from depression to mania. The pattern and associated symptoms often suggest specific psychiatric conditions.

Thought Disorders

Abnormal thought processes may include delusions, hallucinations, or disorganized thinking. The pattern of symptoms often indicates specific psychiatric conditions

Diagnostic procedures

Laboratory studies

Blood Chemistry Analysis

Comprehensive metabolic panels evaluate organ function through measurement of electrolytes, proteins, and metabolic products. These studies assess liver function, kidney function, and metabolic status. Serial measurements often track disease progression and treatment response.

Hematology Studies

Complete blood counts evaluate red cells, white cells, and platelets. Differential white cell counts provide information about infection and inflammation. Coagulation studies assess blood clotting function through various parameters.

Cardiac Enzymes

Specialized blood tests measure markers of cardiac damage. Troponin levels indicate cardiac muscle injury. Additional markers include creatine kinase and myoglobin. Temporal patterns help distinguish acute from chronic cardiac conditions.

Imaging procedures

Radiography

Plain film radiographs provide initial evaluation of various conditions. Chest radiographs assess cardiac and pulmonary status. Skeletal radiographs evaluate bone and joint conditions. Abdominal films identify obstruction or perforation.

Computed Tomography

CT scanning provides detailed cross-sectional imaging. Enhanced studies utilize contrast material for vascular evaluation. Specialized protocols address specific clinical questions. Three-dimensional reconstructions assist surgical planning.

Magnetic Resonance Imaging (MRI)

MRI provides superior soft tissue detail without ionizing radiation. Different scanning sequences highlight specific tissue characteristics. Contrast enhancement identifies areas of inflammation or tumor. Specialized protocols evaluate specific anatomic regions.

Nuclear Medicine

Radioactive tracers evaluate organ function and perfusion. Cardiac studies assess perfusion and function. Bone scans identify areas of increased metabolic activity.

Various protocols address specific diagnostic questions.

Ultrasonography

Sound wave imaging provides real-time evaluation. Cardiac studies assess structure and function. Vascular studies evaluate blood flow patterns. Obstetric studies monitor fetal development.

Table. Common Diagnostic Procedures by System

Body System	Basic Studies	Advanced Studies	Special Procedures
Cardiovascular	ECG, Echo	Stress test	Cardiac catheterization
Respiratory	Spirometry	Chest CT	Bronchoscopy
Gastrointestinal	Basic labs	Endoscopy	ERCP
Neurological	CT scan	MRI	EEG, EMG
Musculoskeletal	X-rays	MRI	Arthroscopy
Endocrine	Blood tests	Nuclear scan	Hormone stimulation tests
Integumentary	Physical exam	Biopsy	Dermoscopy

Cardiovascular studies

Electrocardiography

ECG recordings evaluate cardiac electrical activity. Standard twelve-lead studies provide comprehensive assessment. Continuous monitoring tracks rhythm changes. Exercise testing evaluates cardiac function under stress.

Echocardiography

Cardiac ultrasound evaluates structure and function. Doppler studies assess blood flow patterns. Stress studies evaluate exercise response. Transesophageal studies provide detailed imaging.

Cardiac Catheterization

Direct cardiac chamber assessment through catheter placement. Coronary angiography evaluates vessel patency. Pressure measurements assess valve function. Therapeutic interventions may follow diagnostic studies.

Respiratory studies

Pulmonary Function Testing

Spirometry measures airflow parameters. Lung volume determination assesses static functions. Diffusion capacity evaluates gas exchange. Exercise testing assesses functional capacity.

Bronchoscopy

Direct airway visualization through specialized instruments. Tissue sampling enables pathological diagnosis. Therapeutic interventions may accompany diagnostic procedures.

Gastrointestinal studies

Endoscopy

Direct visualization of gastrointestinal tract. Upper endoscopy examines esophagus, stomach, and duodenum. Colonoscopy examines large intestine. Tissue sampling enables pathological diagnosis.

Radiographic Contrast Studies

Barium studies evaluate gastrointestinal anatomy. Swallowing studies assess upper tract function. Various protocols address specific diagnostic questions.

Neurological studies

Electroencephalography

Brain electrical activity recording through scalp electrodes. Various recording protocols address specific questions. Continuous monitoring evaluates seizure activity.

Nerve Conduction Studies

Peripheral nerve function evaluation through electrical stimulation. Electromyography assesses muscle electrical activity. Combined studies evaluate neuromuscular function.

Musculoskeletal studies

Arthroscopy

Direct joint visualization through specialized instruments. Diagnostic evaluation enables precise diagnosis. Therapeutic interventions may follow diagnostic procedures.

Bone Densitometry

Specialized radiographic assessment of bone density. Various protocols evaluate specific anatomic regions. Serial studies track treatment response.

Urological studies

Cystoscopy

Direct bladder visualization through specialized instruments. Various procedures enable precise diagnosis. Therapeutic interventions may accompany diagnostic studies.

Urodynamics

Specialized testing evaluates bladder function. Pressure measurements assess various parameters. Combined studies evaluate complex conditions.

Gynecological studies

Colposcopy

Detailed cervical examination through specialized instruments. Various techniques enable precise evaluation. Tissue sampling enables pathological diagnosis.

Hysteroscopy

Direct uterine cavity visualization through specialized instruments. Various procedures enable precise diagnosis. Therapeutic interventions may follow diagnostic studies.

Specialized procedures

Biopsy Techniques

Tissue sampling through various approaches. Fine needle aspiration obtains cellular samples. Core biopsies obtain tissue specimens. Surgical biopsies enable complete evaluation.

Diagnostic Aspirations

Fluid sampling from various body cavities. Various techniques address specific situations. Laboratory analysis enables precise diagnosis

TREATMENT MODALITIES

Antimicrobial Therapy

Antibiotics target bacterial infections through various mechanisms. Antiviral medications address specific viral infections. Antifungal agents treat fungal diseases. Selection depends on identified pathogens and resistance patterns.

Cardiovascular Medications

Antihypertensive agents control blood pressure through multiple mechanisms. Anticoagulants prevent thrombotic complications. Antiarrhythmic drugs maintain normal cardiac rhythm. Heart failure medications optimize cardiac function.

Table. Treatment Modalities Overview

Treatment Type	Examples	Primary Applications	Monitoring Requirements
Pharmacological	Antibiotics, Antihypertensives	Infection, Hypertension	Drug levels, Side effects
Surgical	CABG, Joint replacement	CAD, Arthritis	Post-op complications
Physical Therapy	Exercise, Manual therapy	Musculoskeletal conditions	Functional improvement
Radiation	External beam, Brachytherapy	Cancer	Treatment response
Interventional	Angioplasty, Nerve blocks	Vascular disease, Pain	Procedure outcomes
Alternative	Acupuncture, Chiropractic	Various conditions	Symptom improvement
Preventive	Vaccines, Screenings	Disease prevention	Compliance, Results

Respiratory Medications

Bronchodilators improve airflow through various mechanisms. Corticosteroids reduce airway inflammation. Combination therapy addresses multiple disease components. Delivery systems optimize medication effectiveness.

Gastrointestinal Medications

Acid-suppressing agents treat various conditions. Anti-inflammatory medications address bowel disorders. Antiemetics control nausea and vomiting. Prokinetic agents improve gastrointestinal motility.

Endocrine Medications

Diabetes medications regulate blood glucose through various mechanisms. Thyroid medications correct hormonal imbalances. Hormone replacement addresses various deficiency states. Dosing requires careful monitoring and adjustment.

Surgical interventions

Cardiovascular Surgery

Coronary bypass procedures restore blood flow. Valve repairs or replacements correct dysfunction. Aneurysm repairs prevent catastrophic complications. Minimally invasive approaches reduce surgical trauma.

Orthopedic Surgery

Joint replacements restore function. Fracture repairs stabilize injuries. Spinal procedures address various conditions. Arthroscopic techniques enable precise intervention.

Gastrointestinal Surgery

Resection procedures remove diseased segments. Reconstruction restores continuity. Bypass procedures improve function. Minimally invasive approaches reduce recovery time.

Neurological Surgery

Brain tumor resection addresses various lesions. Spinal procedures decompress neural elements. Vascular procedures prevent complications. Stereotactic approaches enable precise intervention.

Therapeutic procedures

Physical Therapy

Exercise programs improve function. Manual techniques address specific conditions. Modalities reduce pain and inflammation. Progressive protocols optimize recovery.

Occupational Therapy

Activities improve daily function. Adaptive techniques enable independence. Environmental modifications optimize safety. Individual programs address specific needs.

Speech Therapy

Communication disorders receive specialized intervention. Swallowing dysfunction requires specific approaches. Cognitive rehabilitation addresses various deficits. Treatment plans reflect individual needs.

Respiratory Therapy

Breathing exercises improve function. Airway clearance techniques prevent complications. Oxygen therapy maintains adequate levels. Equipment selection optimizes effectiveness.

Interventional procedures

Cardiac Catheterization

Angioplasty restores vessel patency. Stent placement maintains improvements. Valve procedures address dysfunction. Various devices address specific conditions.

Radiological Intervention

Image-guided procedures enable precise treatment. Drainage procedures address fluid collections. Vascular interventions restore flow. Various techniques address specific conditions.

Endoscopic Procedures

Therapeutic interventions accompany diagnostic studies. Various techniques address specific conditions. Minimally invasive approaches reduce complications.

Radiation therapy

External Beam Radiation

Precise targeting treats various conditions. Fractionated protocols optimize effectiveness. Side effect management requires careful monitoring. Treatment planning utilizes various imaging modalities.

Brachytherapy

Internal radiation sources treat specific areas. Various techniques address different conditions. Precise placement optimizes effectiveness. Monitoring ensures appropriate dosing.

Rehabilitative services

Cardiac Rehabilitation

Exercise programs improve function. Risk factor modification prevents complications. Education enables self-management. Monitoring ensures safe progression.

Pulmonary Rehabilitation

Breathing exercises improve function. Energy conservation techniques enable activities. Education addresses various aspects. Individual programs reflect specific needs.

Pain management

Medication Protocols

Various agents address different pain types. Combination therapy improves effectiveness. Side effect management requires monitoring. Individual protocols reflect specific needs.

Interventional Techniques

Nerve blocks provide targeted relief. Spinal procedures address various conditions. Device implantation enables long-term management. Various approaches address specific situations.

Alternative therapies

Acupuncture

Traditional techniques address various conditions. Integration with conventional treatment occurs frequently. Various protocols address specific situations. Evidence supports selected applications.

Chiropractic Care

Spinal manipulation addresses various conditions. Additional techniques provide complementary benefits. Integration occurs in various settings. Evidence guides appropriate application.

Preventive care

Immunizations: Vaccination schedules prevent various conditions. Administration follows specific protocols. Documentation requirements ensure compliance. Updates reflect current recommendations.

Screening Programs: Various tests identify early disease. Protocols reflect current guidelines. Documentation supports medical necessity. Follow-up ensures appropriate care.

Summary

Foundational knowledge of human body systems forms the cornerstone of medical coding accuracy. The eleven interconnected organ systems work harmoniously to maintain homeostasis, with each system's function impacting others. Understanding anatomical structures, physiological processes, and system relationships enables coders to accurately identify and code various medical conditions. Common pathologies affecting different body systems demonstrate characteristic patterns, manifestations, and progression, requiring precise documentation and coding. A solid grasp of diagnostic procedures, from basic laboratory tests to advanced imaging studies, helps coders interpret medical records effectively. Knowledge of treatment modalities, including medications, surgical interventions, and therapeutic procedures, ensures appropriate procedure code selection. Familiarity with clinical manifestations across body systems aids in understanding disease processes and their documentation requirements. Integration of preventive care and screening protocols completes the comprehensive approach needed for accurate medical coding.

Multiple Choice Questions

1. Which system serves as the body's first line of defense against external threats?
   a) Immune system
   b) Integumentary system
   c) Muscular system
   d) Nervous system

2. How many bones are present in an adult human body?
   a) 186
   b) 196
   c) 206
   d) 216

3. What percentage of body weight is comprised of skeletal muscles?
   a) 30%
   b) 40%
   c) 50%
   d) 60%

4. The cardiovascular system contains approximately how many miles of blood vessels?
   a) 40,000
   b) 50,000
   c) 60,000
   d) 70,000

5. How many alveoli are present in human lungs?
   a) 100 million
   b) 200 million
   c) 300 million
   d) 400 million

6. How many neurons does the human brain contain approximately?
   a) 66 billion
   b) 76 billion
   c) 86 billion
   d) 96 billion

7. The digestive system spans approximately how many feet in adults?
   a) 20
   b) 25
   c) 30
   d) 35

8. Which condition involves chronic intestinal inflammation?
   a) Peptic ulcer disease
   b) Inflammatory bowel disease
   c) Cirrhosis
   d) Gastritis

9. Type 1 diabetes is characterized by:
   a) Insulin resistance
   b) Insufficient insulin production
   c) Excessive insulin production
   d) Normal insulin levels

10. Which skin cancer demonstrates significant metastatic potential?
    a) Basal cell carcinoma
    b) Squamous cell carcinoma
    c) Melanoma
    d) Actinic keratosis

11. Cardiac-origin chest pain typically presents as:
    a) Sharp, stabbing pain
    b) Burning sensation
    c) Pressure or tightness
    d) Tingling sensation

12. Which is NOT a typical manifestation of heart failure?
    a) Peripheral edema
    b) Dyspnea
    c) Sharp chest pain
    d) Orthopnea

13. What study provides detailed cross-sectional imaging?
    a) Plain radiography
    b) Computed tomography
    c) Ultrasonography
    d) Nuclear medicine

14. Which imaging modality provides superior soft tissue detail without ionizing radiation?
    a) CT scan
    b) X-ray
    c) MRI
    d) Ultrasound

15. ECG recordings evaluate:
    a) Cardiac structure
    b) Blood flow
    c) Electrical activity
    d) Valve function

16. Spirometry measures:
    a) Lung volume

b) Airflow parameters
c) Gas exchange
d) Chest wall movement

17. Direct visualization of the gastrointestinal tract is achieved through:
a) Radiography
b) CT scan
c) Endoscopy
d) Ultrasound

18. Which study evaluates brain electrical activity?
a) EMG
b) EEG
c) ECG
d) NCS

19. Antimicrobial therapy selection depends primarily on:
a) Patient age
b) Cost considerations
c) Identified pathogens and resistance patterns
d) Administration route

20. Which surgical approach reduces recovery time?
a) Open surgery
b) Minimally invasive surgery
c) Traditional surgery
d) Emergency surgery

21. Physical therapy primarily aims to:
a) Prescribe medications
b) Improve function

c) Perform surgery
d) Order diagnostic tests

22. Cardiac catheterization can include:
a) Only diagnostic procedures
b) Only therapeutic procedures
c) Both diagnostic and therapeutic procedures
d) Neither diagnostic nor therapeutic procedures

23. External beam radiation involves:
a) Random targeting
b) Single large dose
c) Precise targeting
d) Internal radiation sources

24. Pain management typically includes:
a) Only medications
b) Only physical therapy
c) Multiple treatment modalities
d) Surgery alone

25. Preventive care includes:
a) Only immunizations
b) Only screening programs
c) Both immunizations and screening programs
d) Neither immunizations nor screening programs

List of Important Questions

1. Explain the interrelationships between major body systems and their significance in medical coding.
2. Describe the structure and function of the integumentary system and common pathologies affecting it.
3. Compare and contrast the skeletal and muscular components of the musculoskeletal system.
4. Analyze the cardiac and vascular components of the cardiovascular system and their clinical significance.
5. Discuss the differences between upper and lower respiratory tract structures and their common pathologies.
6. Explain the central and peripheral nervous system components and their role in body function.
7. Describe common gastrointestinal pathologies and their clinical manifestations.
8. Analyze the pathophysiology and clinical significance of atherosclerosis and hypertension.
9. Compare different types of diagnostic imaging procedures and their applications.
10. Explain the importance of laboratory studies in diagnosis and treatment monitoring.
11. Discuss various cardiovascular diagnostic procedures and their clinical applications.
12. Analyze different treatment modalities for chronic respiratory conditions.
13. Describe common surgical interventions in orthopedic conditions.
14. Explain the role of physical and occupational therapy in patient rehabilitation.
15. Discuss various pain management approaches and their clinical applications.
16. Compare different types of radiation therapy and their therapeutic uses.

17. Analyze the importance of preventive care and screening programs.
18. Describe common endocrine pathologies and their systemic effects.
19. Explain different types of neurological manifestations and their diagnostic significance.
20. Discuss the clinical significance of various hematological disorders.

Bibliography

1. Drake RL, Vogl AW, Mitchell AWM. Gray's Anatomy for Students. 4th ed. Philadelphia: Elsevier; 2020.
2. Kumar V, Abbas AK, Aster JC. Robbins and Cotran Pathologic Basis of Disease. 10th ed. Philadelphia: Elsevier; 2021.
3. Hall JE, Hall ME. Guyton and Hall Textbook of Medical Physiology. 14th ed. Philadelphia: Elsevier; 2020.
4. McPhee SJ, Hammer GD. Pathophysiology of Disease: An Introduction to Clinical Medicine. 8th ed. New York: McGraw-Hill; 2019.
5. Ferri FF. Ferri's Clinical Advisor 2023. Philadelphia: Elsevier; 2023.
6. Goldman L, Schafer AI. Goldman-Cecil Medicine. 26th ed. Philadelphia: Elsevier; 2020.
7. Jameson JL, Fauci AS, Kasper DL, Hauser SL, Longo DL, Loscalzo J. Harrison's Principles of Internal Medicine. 21st ed. New York: McGraw-Hill; 2022.
8. Townsend CM, Beauchamp RD, Evers BM, Mattox KL. Sabiston Textbook of Surgery. 21st ed. Philadelphia: Elsevier; 2022.
9. Bonow RO, Mann DL, Zipes DP, Libby P. Braunwald's Heart Disease. 12th ed. Philadelphia: Elsevier; 2022.
10. Broaddus VC, Ernst JD, King TE, Lazarus SC, Murray JF, Nadel JA. Murray & Nadel's Textbook of Respiratory Medicine. 7th ed. Philadelphia: Elsevier; 2021.
11. Feldman M, Friedman LS, Brandt LJ. Sleisenger and Fordtran's Gastrointestinal and Liver Disease. 11th ed. Philadelphia: Elsevier; 2021.
12. Ropper AH, Samuels MA, Klein JP, Prasad S. Adams and Victor's Principles of Neurology. 12th ed. New York: McGraw-Hill; 2020.
13. Firestein GS, Budd RC, Gabriel SE, McInnes IB,

O'Dell JR. Kelley and Firestein's Textbook of Rheumatology. 11th ed. Philadelphia: Elsevier; 2021.

14. Melmed S, Auchus RJ, Goldfine AB, Koenig RJ, Rosen CJ. Williams Textbook of Endocrinology. 14th ed. Philadelphia: Elsevier; 2020.
15. Hoffman R, Benz EJ, Silberstein LE, Heslop HE, Weitz JI, Anastasi J. Hematology: Basic Principles and Practice. 7th ed. Philadelphia: Elsevier; 2018.
16. Bolognia JL, Schaffer JV, Cerroni L. Dermatology. 4th ed. Philadelphia: Elsevier; 2018.
17. Kasper DL, Fauci AS, Hauser SL, Longo DL, Jameson JL, Loscalzo J. Harrison's Manual of Medicine. 20th ed. New York: McGraw-Hill; 2020.
18. Goldman L, Schafer AI. Goldman's Cecil Medicine. 26th ed. Philadelphia: Elsevier; 2020.
19. Brunicardi FC, Andersen DK, Billiar TR, Dunn DL, Hunter JG, Matthews JB, et al. Schwartz's Principles of Surgery. 11th ed. New York: McGraw-Hill; 2019.
20. Kumar P, Clark M. Kumar and Clark's Clinical Medicine. 10th ed. Philadelphia: Elsevier; 2020.

CHAPTER 5

NAVIGATION AND CODE LOCATION

Author

Mr. Prakash Nathaniel Kumar Sarella, Associate Professor, Department of Pharmaceutics, Aditya College of Pharmacy, Aditya University, Surampalem, Andhra Pradesh, India

Abstract

The ICD-10-CM manual is structured as a comprehensive diagnostic coding system with multiple organizational components designed for efficient code location and accurate assignment. The manual's front matter includes essential instructional notes, conventions, and guidelines, followed by an alphabetically organized index. The tabular list comprises twenty-one chapters organized by body systems, with additional chapters for special circumstances. Codes follow an alphanumeric structure where the first three characters identify broad categories, while subsequent characters provide greater specificity. The manual employs various navigation aids including color coding, page headers, and margin notes to facilitate quick reference. Supplementary sections contain appendices and drug tables for additional reference. The Index to Diseases and Injuries follows an alphabetical organization with main terms and indented subterms, reflecting clinical terminology and anatomical relationships. The manual undergoes annual revisions and quarterly electronic updates to maintain currency with medical knowledge and coding requirements. Code format maintains consistency throughout, with specific notation systems for includes/excludes notes, sequencing guidance, and encounter types. The hierarchical structure progresses from general to specific concepts, with modifiers and anatomical specifications providing increasing levels of detail.

Keywords: *Alphanumeric coding system; Diagnostic classification; Hierarchical organization; Clinical terminology; Tabular indexing*

Learning Objectives

After completion of the chapter, the learners should be able to:

- Identify the major sections of the ICD-10-CM manual and explain their purpose in the coding process.
- Demonstrate proper use of the manual's navigation aids, including color coding, page headers, and margin notes.
- Analyze the structure of diagnostic codes, including the significance of character positions and notation systems.
- Utilize the Index to Diseases and Injuries effectively by understanding main term entries, subterm arrangements, and cross-references.
- Interpret instructional notes, including includes/excludes notes and code first guidelines, to ensure accurate code assignment.
- Recognize the update cycle of the ICD-10-CM manual and understand the implementation of annual revisions and quarterly modifications.

ICD-10-CM MANUAL ORGANIZATION

Volume Organization

The ICD-10-CM manual consists of multiple sections designed for systematic code location. The Table of Contents provides initial navigation guidance. The Preface contains vital usage information. The Coding Guidelines offer essential instruction for proper code assignment.

Classification System

The diagnostic codes follow an alphanumeric system

structure. Each chapter addresses specific condition categories. Codes progress from general to specific concepts. Organization reflects anatomical systems and disease processes.

Table. ICD-10-CM Manual Section Organization

Section	Primary Function	Components
Front Matter	Orientation and Guidance	Table of Contents Preface Coding Guidelines
Index to Diseases	Code Location	Alphabetic Listings Main Terms Subterms
Tabular List	Code Selection	21 Body Systems Special Chapters Code Categories
Appendices	Supplementary Information	Drug Tables Reference Materials Special Guidelines

Front matter

Instructional Notes

The manual begins with comprehensive usage instructions. Conventions explain standardized notation systems. General guidelines address overarching coding principles. Chapter-specific guidelines provide detailed direction.

Index Information

Alphabetic organization facilitates initial code location. Main terms lead to more specific subterms. Cross-references guide users to appropriate entries.

Notation systems indicate special coding requirements.

Tabular list

Chapter Structure

Twenty-one chapters organize conditions by body system. Additional chapters address special circumstances. Each chapter contains related condition categories. Organization follows logical disease progression.

Code Categories

Three-character categories represent broad concepts. Additional characters provide greater specificity. Hierarchical organization guides code selection. Related conditions appear in proximity.

Section Headers

Bold headers identify major code sections. Subheadings indicate specific condition groups. Hierarchical organization guides navigation. Visual cues facilitate quick reference.

Code format

Basic Structure

Characters one through three identify the category. Characters four through six provide additional detail. Character seven indicates encounter type when applicable. Format remains consistent throughout the manual.

Code Components

The first character appears as a letter. Characters two through seven appear as numbers. Decimal points separate third and fourth characters. Precise positioning carries specific meaning.

Special Notations

Includes notes identify related conditions. Excludes notes prevent incorrect code assignment. Code first notes guide sequencing decisions. Additional notes provide specific instruction.

Table. Code Character Positions and Their Meanings

Character Position	Format	Purpose	Example
1st	Letter	Category identification	M - Musculoskeletal
2nd-3rd	Number	Category specification	M16 - Osteoarthritis of hip
4th	Number	Etiology, anatomic site	M16.1 - Unilateral primary OA
5th-6th	Number	Additional specificity	M16.12 - Left hip OA
7th	Number	Encounter type	M16.12A - Initial encounter

Navigation aids

Color Coding

Different colors identify distinct sections. Visual cues facilitate quick reference. Consistent application aids navigation. Color schemes remain standard throughout editions.

Page Headers

Running headers identify current sections. Page numbers enable precise location. Chapter references maintain orientation. Quick reference facilitation occurs throughout.

Margin Notes

Side notes provide additional information. Quick reference aids appear when needed. Notation systems remain consistent. Important points receive emphasis.

Supplementary sections

Appendices

Additional information appears in appendices. Various topics receive detailed coverage. Reference materials provide support. Location follows the main code sections.

Drug Tables

Medication-related information appears separately. Organization facilitates quick reference. Cross-references guide appropriate usage. Updates reflect current standards.

Table. Navigation Tools and Their Functions

Navigation Tool	Location	Purpose	Usage Tips
Color Coding	Throughout manual	Section identification	Match colors for related sections
Page Headers	Top of each page	Location orientation	Shows current chapter/section
Section Dividers	Between major sections	Quick access	Use tabs for frequent sections
Margin Notes	Side of pages	Additional information	Check for special instructions
Running Headers	Throughout manual	Current content reference	Use for rapid navigation
Cross-References	Within content	Alternative term location	Follow "see" and "see also" notes

Coding tools

Section Dividers

Physical dividers separate major sections. Quick access enables efficient navigation. Labeled tabs identify contents. Organization reflects frequent usage patterns.

Highlighting Systems

Color coding identifies important information. Consistent systems enhance efficiency. Personal notation adds value. Organization remains individually relevant.

Manual updates

Annual Revisions

Updates reflect current medical knowledge. Changes appear in various sections. Documentation explains modifications. Implementation follows specific schedules.

Quarterly Updates

Electronic versions receive frequent updates. Changes reflect current requirements. Documentation explains modifications. Implementation follows specific schedules.

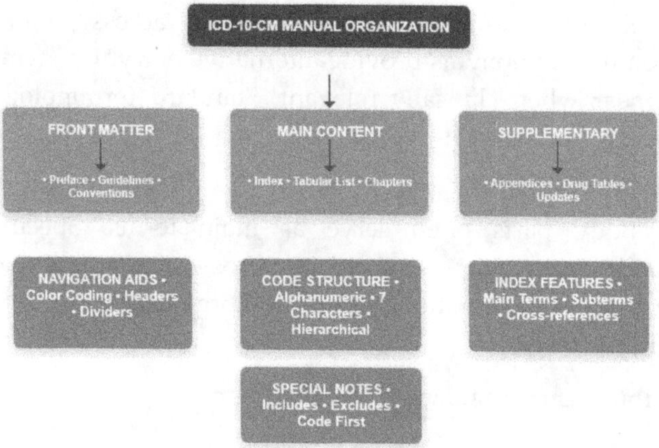

INDEX TO DISEASES AND INJURIES

Index structure

Alphabetical Organization

Main terms appear in alphabetical sequence. Indented subterms provide additional specificity. Cross-references guide alternative term locations. Organization facilitates systematic code location.

Entry Format

Main terms appear in bold type. Modifying terms appear indented below. Essential modifiers affect code selection. Format remains consistent throughout.

Main term entries

Primary Terms

Disease names serve as primary access points. Common synonyms provide alternative entry. Eponyms appear when clinically relevant. Standard terminology receives preference.

Anatomical Sites

Body parts often serve as main terms. Specific conditions appear as subentries. Cross-references guide appropriate navigation. Anatomical organization reflects clinical usage.

Subterm arrangement

Hierarchical Structure: Indentation indicates relationship levels. More specific terms appear beneath main terms. Multiple levels provide increasing detail. Organization reflects clinical terminology.

Modifier Sequence: Essential modifiers appear first. Secondary characteristics follow. Temporal factors affect code selection. Location specifics complete descriptions.

Summary

The ICD-10-CM manual organization follows a structured approach to facilitate efficient code location and accurate assignment. The manual's architecture includes front matter containing essential guidelines, an alphabetic index, and a tabular list organized by body systems. The code format employs an alphanumeric system where characters hold specific meaning and position significance. Navigation is enhanced through color coding, page headers, and margin notes, while supplementary sections provide additional reference materials. The Index to Diseases and Injuries maintains an alphabetical structure with main terms and subterms arranged hierarchically to reflect clinical relationships. Regular updates through annual revisions and quarterly electronic modifications ensure the manual remains current with medical knowledge and coding requirements.

Multiple Choice Questions

1. Which section of the ICD-10-CM manual provides initial navigation guidance?
   a) Preface
   b) Table of Contents
   c) Coding Guidelines
   d) Tabular List

2. How many chapters organize conditions by body system in ICD-10-CM?
   a) 19
   b) 20
   c) 21
   d) 22

3. The first character in an ICD-10-CM code appears as a:
   a) Number
   b) Letter
   c) Symbol
   d) Decimal point

4. What separates the third and fourth characters in an ICD-10-CM code?
   a) Hyphen
   b) Space
   c) Decimal point
   d) Comma

5. Electronic versions of ICD-10-CM receive updates:
   a) Monthly
   b) Quarterly
   c) Annually
   d) Bi-annually

6. In the Index to Diseases and Injuries, main terms appear in:
   a) Italic type
   b) Bold type
   c) Regular type
   d) Underlined type

7. The seventh character in an ICD-10-CM code typically indicates:
   a) Diagnosis type
   b) Encounter type
   c) Body system
   d) Location specifics

8. Which notes prevent incorrect code assignment?
   a) Includes notes
   b) Code first notes
   c) Excludes notes
   d) Additional notes

9. Characters four through six in an ICD-10-CM code provide:
   a) Category information
   b) Additional detail
   c) Encounter type
   d) Body system

10. The Index to Diseases and Injuries is organized:
    a) Numerically
    b) By body system
    c) Alphabetically
    d) Chronologically

11. Which manual section contains vital usage information?
    a) Table of Contents
    b) Preface
    c) Index
    d) Appendices

12. Main terms in the index lead to:
    a) More specific subterms
    b) Chapter numbers
    c) Color codes
    d) Page headers

13. Bold headers in the Tabular List identify:
    a) Page numbers
    b) Major code sections

c) Cross-references
d) Drug tables

14. The manual's organization reflects:
a) Administrative preferences
b) Alphabetical order
c) Anatomical systems and disease processes
d) Publishing standards

15. Margin notes in the manual provide:
a) Page numbers
b) Additional information
c) Chapter titles
d) Color codes

16. The classification system structure is:
a) Numeric
b) Alphabetic
c) Alphanumeric
d) Symbolic

17. Cross-references in the index guide users to:
a) Page numbers
b) Appropriate entries
c) Color codes
d) Chapter titles

18. Essential modifiers in code selection appear:
a) Last
b) First
c) Randomly
d) Alphabetically

19. The manual's code categories progress from:
a) Specific to general

b) General to specific
c) Simple to complex
d) Complex to simple

20. Running headers help identify:
 a) Current sections
 b) Code numbers
 c) Drug information
 d) Updates

21. Indentation in the index indicates:
 a) Page breaks
 b) New chapters
 c) Relationship levels
 d) Code changes

22. Characters one through three identify the:
 a) Encounter type
 b) Body system
 c) Category
 d) Specificity

23. The manual's highlighting system is designed to:
 a) Enhance efficiency
 b) Save space
 c) Add color
 d) Mark errors

24. Anatomical sites in the index appear as:
 a) Appendices
 b) Main terms
 c) Footnotes
 d) Headers

25. The manual's supplementary sections appear:
    a) Before the main code sections
    b) Within the main code sections
    c) Following the main code sections
    d) Throughout the manual

List of Important Questions

1. What is the fundamental organization structure of the ICD-10-CM manual and how does it facilitate code location?
2. Describe the hierarchical arrangement of codes and explain how it contributes to accurate code selection.
3. How do instructional notes in ICD-10-CM guide proper code assignment? Discuss the different types.
4. Explain the significance of the seven-character code structure in ICD-10-CM.
5. Compare and contrast the roles of the Alphabetic Index and the Tabular List.
6. What is the purpose of color coding in the ICD-10-CM manual and how does it enhance navigation?
7. Discuss the importance of includes and excludes notes in code assignment.
8. How do quarterly updates differ from annual revisions in the ICD-10-CM manual?
9. Explain the relationship between main terms and subterms in the Index to Diseases and Injuries.
10. What role do cross-references play in the coding process?
11. Describe the significance of anatomical site organization in the manual.
12. How do page headers and margin notes contribute to efficient manual navigation?
13. Explain the purpose and organization of the supplementary sections.
14. What is the role of the preface and coding guidelines in proper code assignment?
15. Describe how modifier sequences affect code selection.
16. How does the manual's organization reflect clinical terminology and practice?

17. Explain the significance of the decimal point placement in ICD-10-CM codes.
18. What is the purpose of code first notes and how do they affect sequencing?
19. Describe the relationship between the Table of Contents and efficient code location.
20. How do appendices and drug tables support the coding process?

Bibliography

1. Bowman S. Coordination of SNOMED-CT and ICD-10: getting the most out of electronic health record systems. Perspect Health Inf Manag. 2005;2:7.
2. Butler R. ICD-10 implementation: a primer for healthcare providers. J AHIMA. 2016;87(2):36-41.
3. Centers for Medicare & Medicaid Services. ICD-10-CM Official Guidelines for Coding and Reporting FY 2024. Baltimore: CMS; 2023.
4. Steindel SJ. International classification of diseases, 10th edition, clinical modification and procedure coding system: descriptive overview of the next generation HIPAA code sets. J Am Med Inform Assoc. 2010;17(3):274-82.
5. O'Malley KJ, Cook KF, Price MD, et al. Measuring diagnoses: ICD code accuracy. Health Serv Res. 2005;40(5):1620-39.
6. Manchikanti L, Falco FJ, Hirsch JA. Necessity and implications of ICD-10: facts and fallacies. Pain Physician. 2011;14(5):E405-25.
7. Giannangelo K, Hyde L. Breaking down the code: ICD-10-CM diagnosis codes. J AHIMA. 2012;83(11):52-4.
8. Quan H, Sundararajan V, Halfon P, et al. Coding algorithms for defining comorbidities in ICD-9-CM and ICD-10 administrative data. Med Care. 2005;43(11):1130-9.
9. World Health Organization. International Statistical Classification of Diseases and Related Health Problems, 10th Revision. Geneva: WHO; 2019.
10. Sanders TB, Bowens FM, Pierce W, et al. The road to ICD-10-CM/PCS implementation: forecasting the transition for providers. Perspect Health Inf Manag. 2012;9:1f.

11. Topaz M, Shafran-Topaz L, Bowles KH. ICD-10: transitions for healthcare providers. Prof Case Manag. 2013;18(4):186-96.
12. Manchikanti L, Falco FJ, Hirsch JA. Ready or not! Here comes ICD-10. J Neurointerv Surg. 2013;5(1):86-91.
13. Cassidy A. Health policy brief: implementing ICD-10. Health Aff (Millwood). 2014;33(2):1-5.
14. Meyer H. Coding complexity: US healthcare gets ready for ICD-10. Health Aff (Millwood). 2011;30(5):968-74.
15. Januel JM, Luthi JC, Quan H, et al. Improved accuracy of co-morbidity coding over time after the introduction of ICD-10 administrative data. BMC Health Serv Res. 2011;11:194.
16. DeAlmeida DR, Watzlaf VJ, Anania-Firouzan P, et al. Evaluation of inpatient clinical documentation readiness for ICD-10-CM. Perspect Health Inf Manag. 2014;11:1h.
17. Manchikanti L, Hirsch JA. Ready or not! Here comes ICD-10. J Neurointerv Surg. 2013;5(1):86-91.
18. Utter GH, Cox GL, Owens PL, Romano PS. Challenges and opportunities with ICD-10-CM/PCS. J AHIMA. 2013;84(7):70-1.
19. Weems S, Heller P, Fenton SH. Results from the Veterans Health Administration ICD-10-CM/PCS coding pilot study. Perspect Health Inf Manag. 2015;12:1b.
20. Ross-Davis SV. Preparing for ICD-10-CM/PCS implementation: impact on productivity and quality. Perspect Health Inf Manag. 2012;9:1f.

CHAPTER 6

CODING BY BODY SYSTEM

Author

Mr. Rajasekhar Bariki, Associate professor, Dept. of Pharmaceutics, St Johns College of Pharmaceutical Sciences, Yerrakota, Kurnool, Andhra Pradesh

Abstract

The ICD-10-CM coding system organizes diseases and conditions across major body systems, providing detailed classification for medical coding and billing. Chapters span infectious diseases, neoplasms, endocrine disorders, mental health, neurological conditions, circulatory system diseases, respiratory conditions, digestive disorders, musculoskeletal problems, genitourinary diseases, pregnancy/childbirth, and skin conditions. Each chapter includes specific code ranges with detailed subcategories for precise condition identification. Documentation requirements emphasize specificity in anatomical location, disease type, acuity, severity, causative factors, and associated manifestations. Key coding guidelines address proper sequencing, combination code usage, and additional code requirements for complete diagnostic representation. Multiple code scenarios require attention to underlying conditions, complications, and treatment status. Special documentation elements include staging information, risk factors, clinical indicators, and treatment responses. The system requires thorough clinical documentation to support accurate code assignment across all body systems, with particular emphasis on causal relationships, manifestations, and clinical specificity.

Keywords: *ICD-10-CM; Medical coding; Clinical documentation; Disease classification; Diagnostic specificity*

Learning Objectives

After completion of the chapter, the student should be able to:

- Demonstrate proficiency in navigating the ICD-10-CM classification system across major body systems and disease categories
- Apply coding guidelines correctly for condition type, anatomical location, severity, and manifestations
- Identify necessary documentation elements required for accurate code assignment in different disease categories
- Understand proper sequencing rules and combination code usage for complex medical conditions
- Recognize when multiple codes are needed to fully represent a patient's diagnostic picture
- Evaluate clinical documentation for completeness and specificity to support accurate code selection

INFECTIOUS AND PARASITIC DISEASES

Intestinal infections (A00-A09)

Includes infections caused by organisms affecting the gastrointestinal tract. Common conditions like cholera (A00), typhoid fever (A01), and salmonella infections (A02) fall in this range. Key manifestations and complications determine specific code selection.

Tuberculosis (A15-A19)

Covers respiratory TB (A15) and TB affecting other body systems (A18). Documentation must specify:

- Bacteriological confirmation

- Affected sites
- Manifestations
- Treatment status

Bacterial diseases (A20-A49)

Major category includes sepsis (A40-A41), bacterial infections, and their complications. Important distinctions:

- Causative organism
- Site of infection
- Associated manifestations
- Resistance patterns (like MRSA)

Viral infections (B00-B34)

Encompasses herpes viral infections (B00), viral hepatitis (B15-B19), and HIV disease (B20). Key coding considerations:

- Virus type
- Acute vs chronic
- Manifestations
- Current status

Mycoses (B35-B49)

Fungal infections affecting various body sites, including:

- Dermatophytosis (B35)
- Candidiasis (B37)
- Other fungal infections Site specificity and systemic involvement guide code selection.

Parasitic diseases (B50-B89)

Includes conditions like malaria (B50-B54) and other parasitic infections. Documentation should specify:

- Parasite type
- Affected systems
- Complications
- Treatment response

Other infectious diseases (B90-B99)

Covers sequelae of previous infections and late effects. Important to document:

- Original condition
- Current manifestations
- Causal relationship

Coding guidelines

1. Sequence based on circumstances of admission
2. Include manifestation codes when applicable
3. Document infectious agent when known
4. Specify acute vs chronic status
5. Note any drug resistance
6. Include treatment status

Table. Commonly Used Infectious Disease Codes and Documentation Requirements

Disease Category	Code Range	Essential Documentation	Required Specifics
Tuberculosis	A15-A19	Site, Bacteriology, Treatment	Culture results, Response
Sepsis	A40-A41	Causative organism, Severity	Acute organ dysfunction
Viral hepatitis	B15-B19	Type, Chronicity, Carrier status	Serological markers
HIV disease	B20	Stage, CD4 count, Manifestations	Current medications
Mycoses	B35-B49	Location, Type, Severity	Culture confirmation

NEOPLASMS

Malignant Neoplasms (C00-C96)

Primary sites organized by anatomical location:

- Head/Neck (C00-C14): Lip, oral cavity, pharynx
- Digestive System (C15-C26): Esophagus to rectum
- Respiratory System (C30-C39): Nasal cavity to lung
- Bone/Cartilage (C40-C41)
- Skin (C43-C44): Melanoma vs other skin cancers
- Soft Tissue (C45-C49)
- Breast (C50)
- Female Organs (C51-C58)
- Male Organs (C60-C63)
- Urinary System (C64-C68)
- CNS/Endocrine (C69-C75)
- Blood/Lymphatic (C81-C96)

Secondary Malignancies (C77-C79)

Metastatic sites:

- Lymph nodes (C77)
- Respiratory/digestive organs (C78)
- Other specified sites (C79)

Benign Neoplasms (D10-D36)

Organized by anatomical site:

- Oral/digestive (D10-D13)
- Respiratory/intrathoracic (D14-D15)
- Bone/connective tissue (D16-D17)
- Soft tissue (D18-D21)
- Reproductive system (D25-D28)
- Urinary system (D29-D30)
- CNS/endocrine (D32-D35)

UNCERTAIN BEHAVIOR/UNSPECIFIED (D37-D49)

Used when behavior (malignant vs benign) is unclear:

- Digestive/respiratory (D37-D38)
- Reproductive (D39-D41)
- Other sites (D42-D48)
- Unspecified sites (D49)

CODING GUIDELINES:

1. Primary Site Documentation:
- Exact location
- Laterality when applicable
- Morphological type
- Behavior (malignant/benign)
2. Required Information:
- Current vs historical
- Active treatment status
- Metastatic sites
- Remission status
3. Sequencing Rules:
- Current treatment: primary site first
- Metastasis treatment: secondary site first
- Complications: sequence based on circumstances
4. Additional Codes Needed For:
- Treatment complications
- Associated conditions
- Functional activity
- Personal history

Remember: Always verify histological confirmation and current status before code assignment.

Table. Neoplasm Classification and Coding Requirements

Site	Malignant Primary	Malignant Secondary	Benign	Documentation Needs
Breast	C50	C79.81	D24	Laterality, Histology
Lung	C34	C78.0	D14.3	Location, Type
Colon	C18	C78.5	D12	Specific segment
Prostate	C61	C79.82	D29.1	PSA, Gleason score
Skin	C43-C44	C79.2	D23	Morphology, Site

ENDOCRINE AND METABOLIC DISORDERS

Thyroid disorders (E00-E07)

Includes disorders affecting thyroid function:

- Iodine deficiency disorders (E00-E02)
- Hypothyroidism (E03)
- Hyperthyroidism/thyrotoxicosis (E05)
- Thyroiditis (E06)
- Other thyroid disorders (E07)

Diabetes mellitus (E08-E13)

Types and complications:

- Type 1 diabetes (E10)
- Type 2 diabetes (E11)
- Secondary diabetes (E08, E09, E13)

Common complications require additional digits for:

- Kidney complications
- Ophthalmic complications
- Neurological complications

- Circulatory complications
- Other specified complications

Obesity and nutritional disorders (E65-E68)

Includes:

- Localized adiposity (E65)
- Obesity (E66)
- Other hyperalimentation (E67-E68)

Metabolic disorders (E70-E88)

Covers disorders of:

- Amino acid metabolism (E70-E72)
- Carbohydrate metabolism (E73-E74)
- Lipid metabolism (E75-E76)
- Purine/pyrimidine metabolism (E79)
- Mineral metabolism (E83)
- Fluid/electrolyte balance (E86-E87)

Other endocrine Disorders (E20-E35)

Including:

- Parathyroid disorders (E20-E21)
- Pituitary disorders (E22-E23)
- Adrenal gland disorders (E24-E27)
- Ovarian/testicular dysfunction (E28-E29)
- Multiple endocrine disorders (E31)

Coding guidelines:

Diabetes Documentation Needs:

- Type
- Control status
- Complications
- Treatment regimen

Important Details:

- Underlying causes

- Associated manifestations
- Acute vs chronic
- Treatment status

Combination Codes:

- Use when available
- Include manifestations
- Note causal relationships

Additional Coding:

- Long-term medication use
- Secondary conditions
- Complications of treatment
- BMI when relevant

MENTAL HEALTH CONDITIONS

Includes conditions affecting cognitive function:

- Vascular dementia (F01)
- Dementia in other diseases (F02)
- Unspecified dementia (F03)
- Delirium (F05)
- Other mental disorders due to physiological conditions (F06-F09)

Substance-related disorders (F10-F19)

Organized by substance type:

- Alcohol (F10)
- Opioids (F11)
- Cannabis (F12)
- Sedatives/hypnotics (F13)
- Cocaine (F14)
- Other stimulants (F15)
- Hallucinogens (F16)

Common fourth/fifth digits indicate:

- Use
- Dependence
- Withdrawal
- Psychotic disorders
- Sleep disorders
- Mood disorders

Schizophrenia and Psychotic Disorders (F20-F29)

Major categories include:

- Schizophrenia (F20)
- Schizotypal disorder (F21)
- Delusional disorders (F22)
- Brief psychotic disorder (F23)
- Schizoaffective disorders (F25)

Mood disorders (F30-F39)

Includes:

- Bipolar disorders (F31)
- Major depressive disorder (F32-F33)
- Persistent mood disorders (F34)
- Other mood disorders (F38-F39)

Anxiety and stress-related disorders (F40-F48)

Categories cover:

- Phobic anxiety disorders (F40)
- Panic disorder (F41.0)
- Generalized anxiety (F41.1)
- OCD (F42)
- PTSD/Adjustment disorders (F43)

Behavioral syndromes (F50-F59)

Including:

- Eating disorders (F50)

- Sleep disorders (F51)
- Sexual dysfunction (F52)

Coding guidelines:

Documentation Requirements:

- Specific disorder type
- Severity level
- Episode status
- Remission status
- Associated manifestations

Main Considerations:

- Acute vs chronic
- Treatment status
- Therapeutic response
- Comorbid conditions

Multiple Coding Rules:

- Underlying conditions
- Manifestations
- Substance use involvement
- Medical complications

Special Attention:

- Suicide risk status
- Violence risk factors
- Legal status
- Treatment compliance

Remember:

- Code to highest specificity
- Include status indicators
- Document behavioral manifestations
- Note treatment modalities

NERVOUS SYSTEM DISORDERS

Central nervous system infections (G00-G09)

Includes inflammatory conditions:

- Bacterial meningitis (G00)
- Meningitis in other diseases (G01-G02)
- Encephalitis/myelitis (G04-G05)
- Intracranial/intraspinal abscess (G06-G07)
- Post-infectious conditions (G09)

Degenerative diseases (G10-G14)

Primary conditions:

- Huntington's disease (G10)
- Parkinson's disease (G20)
- Alzheimer's disease (G30)
- Motor neuron disease/ALS (G12)
- Multiple sclerosis (G35)

Movement disorders (G20-G26)

Including:

- Parkinsonism (G20-G22)
- Dystonia (G24)
- Essential tremor (G25)
- Extrapyramidal disorders (G25)

Epilepsy and seizures (G40-G47)

Types and manifestations:

- Focal epilepsy (G40.0-G40.1)
- Generalized epilepsy (G40.3)
- Status epilepticus (G41)
- Migraine (G43)
- Other headache syndromes (G44)
- Sleep disorders (G47)

Nerve/nerve root disorders (G50-G59)

Conditions affecting:

- Cranial nerves (G50-G53)

- Nerve roots/plexuses (G54)
- Mononeuropathies (G56-G58)
- Polyneuropathy (G60-G65)

Muscular and neuromuscular disorders (G70-G73)

Including:

- Myasthenia gravis (G70)
- Muscular dystrophy (G71)
- Periodic paralysis (G72)
- Other myopathies (G73)

Coding guidelines:

Essential Documentation:

- Specific condition/type
- Acute vs chronic
- Severity level
- Manifestations
- Treatment status

Key Components:

- Underlying causes
- Associated symptoms
- Neurological deficits
- Treatment response

Multiple Code Requirements:

- Manifestation codes
- Causal conditions
- Complications
- Secondary effects

Special Considerations:

- Status indicators
- Functional impact
- Treatment complications
- Recovery status

CIRCULATORY SYSTEM

Hypertensive diseases (I10-I16)

Types and complications:

- Essential hypertension (I10)
- Hypertensive heart disease (I11)
- Hypertensive kidney disease (I12)
- Hypertensive heart and kidney disease (I13)
- Secondary hypertension (I15)
- Hypertensive crisis (I16)

Ischemic Heart Disease (I20-I25)

Includes:

- Angina pectoris (I20)
- Acute myocardial infarction (I21)
- Subsequent myocardial infarction (I22)
- Chronic ischemic heart disease (I25)
- Coronary artery disease

Heart failure (I50)

Types specified as:

- Systolic (reduced ejection fraction)
- Diastolic (preserved ejection fraction)
- Combined systolic and diastolic
- Acute, chronic, or acute on chronic

Cardiac Arrhythmias (I47-I49)

Including:

- Atrial fibrillation/flutter (I48)
- Ventricular tachycardia (I47)
- Heart blocks (I44-I45)
- Other conduction disorders

Cerebrovascular Diseases (I60-I69)

Categories include:

- Subarachnoid hemorrhage (I60)
- Intracerebral hemorrhage (I61)
- Cerebral infarction (I63)
- Stroke sequelae (I69)
- TIA (G45)

Vascular diseases (I70-I79)

Covering:

- Atherosclerosis (I70)
- Aortic aneurysm (I71)
- Peripheral vascular disease (I73)
- Arterial embolism/thrombosis (I74)

Venous conditions (I80-I89)

Including:

- Deep vein thrombosis (I82)
- Varicose veins (I83)
- Chronic venous insufficiency (I87)
- Phlebitis/thrombophlebitis (I80)

Coding guidelines:

Documentation Requirements:

- Acuity (acute/chronic)
- Type/location
- Severity
- Causative factors
- Associated complications

Combination Codes:

- Hypertension with heart disease
- Hypertension with kidney disease
- Atherosclerosis with complications

- Heart failure type and acuity

Sequencing Rules:

- Principal diagnosis selection
- Multiple condition coding
- Complications
- Underlying causes

Special Attention:

- Current vs historical
- Treatment status
- Risk factors
- Manifestations

Clinical Indicators Needed:

- Diagnostic test results
- Clinical findings
- Treatment responses
- Status changes

Table. Cardiovascular Conditions Coding Matrix

Condition	Primary Code	Additional Codes Required	Documentation
HTN with Heart Disease	I11.0-I11.9	Heart failure type if present	EF%, Symptoms
Acute MI	I21.0-I21.9	Location, Initial vs Subsequent	EKG, Enzymes
Heart Failure	I50.1-I50.9	Systolic vs Diastolic	EF%, NYHA class
Atrial Fibrillation	I48.0-I48.9	Chronic vs Paroxysmal	Type, Treatment
CAD	I25.10-I25.119	Vessel involvement	Stenosis %, Symptoms

RESPIRATORY SYSTEM

Acute Upper Respiratory Infections (J00-J06)

Common conditions:

- Acute nasopharyngitis/cold (J00)
- Acute sinusitis (J01)
- Acute pharyngitis (J02)
- Acute tonsillitis (J03)
- Acute laryngitis/tracheitis (J04)
- Upper respiratory infections of multiple sites (J06)

Influenza and pneumonia (J09-J18)

Categories include:

- Influenza due to identified virus (J09-J11)
- Viral pneumonia (J12)
- Bacterial pneumonia (J13-J15)
- Pneumonia due to other organisms (J16)
- Pneumonia, unspecified organism (J18)

Chronic lower respiratory diseases (J40-J47)

Including:

- Bronchitis (J40-J42)
- Emphysema (J43)
- COPD (J44)
- Asthma (J45)
- Status asthmaticus (J46)
- Bronchiectasis (J47)

Other respiratory conditions (J30-J39)

Covering:

- Allergic rhinitis (J30)
- Chronic rhinitis/sinusitis (J31-J32)
- Nasal polyps (J33)

- Diseases of vocal cords/larynx (J38)

Lung diseases due to external agents (J60-J70)

Including:

- Pneumoconiosis (J60-J65)
- Airway disease due to specific dust
- Hypersensitivity pneumonitis (J67)
- Respiratory conditions due to chemicals/fumes (J68)

Respiratory failure (J96)

Types specified as:

- Acute
- Chronic
- Acute on chronic
- With hypoxia/hypercapnia

Coding guidelines:

Documentation Requirements:

- Acuity (acute/chronic)
- Causative organism if known
- Associated conditions
- Tobacco use/exposure
- Severity indicators

Key Components:

- Type of condition
- Underlying causes
- Complications
- Treatment response

Combination Coding:

- Infectious agents
- Manifestations
- Tobacco-related conditions
- Environmental factors

Important Indicators:

- Oxygen dependency
- Respiratory support
- Exercise tolerance
- Acute exacerbations

Clinical Documentation Needs:

- Pulmonary function tests
- Blood gas results
- Imaging findings
- Response to therapy

DIGESTIVE SYSTEM

Oral cavity and salivary glands (K00-K14)

Including:

- Disorders of tooth development (K00)
- Dental caries (K02)
- Periodontal diseases (K05)
- Stomatitis/oral lesions (K12)
- Diseases of salivary glands (K11)
- Diseases of tongue (K14)

Esophagus, stomach, duodenum (K20-K31)

Conditions including:

- Esophagitis (K20)
- GERD (K21)
- Gastric ulcer (K25)
- Duodenal ulcer (K26)
- Gastritis/duodenitis (K29)
- Other disorders (K31)

Intestinal Diseases (K50-K64)

Major categories:

- Crohn's disease (K50)
- Ulcerative colitis (K51)
- IBS (K58)
- Intestinal malabsorption (K90)
- Diverticular disease (K57)
- Hemorrhoids (K64)

Liver diseases (K70-K77)

Including:

- Alcoholic liver disease (K70)
- Toxic liver disease (K71)
- Hepatic failure (K72)
- Chronic hepatitis (K73)
- Fibrosis/cirrhosis (K74)
- Other liver disorders (K76)

Biliary tract/pancreas (K80-K87)

Covering:

- Cholelithiasis (K80)
- Cholecystitis (K81)
- Acute pancreatitis (K85)
- Chronic pancreatitis (K86)
- Other disorders (K87)

Coding guidelines:

Documentation Requirements:

- Acuity (acute/chronic)
- Site specificity
- Causative factors
- Complications
- Bleeding status

Key Components:

- Location
- Severity
- Associated conditions
- Treatment response
- Manifestations

Multiple Code Considerations:

- Underlying conditions
- Manifestations
- Complications
- Associated symptoms

Special Documentation:

- Bleeding status
- Alcohol involvement
- Infection presence
- Obstruction status

Important Clinical Indicators:

- Laboratory findings
- Imaging results
- Endoscopic findings
- Surgical findings

Remember to Document:

- Specific anatomical sites
- Causative organisms
- Treatment outcomes
- Risk factors

Attention Required for:

- Acute vs chronic status
- Severity indicators
- Complication presence
- Treatment response

MUSCULOSKELETAL SYSTEM

Arthropathies (M00-M25)

Infectious and inflammatory:

- Infectious arthritis (M00-M02)
- Rheumatoid arthritis (M05-M06)
- Psoriatic arthritis (M07)
- Gout (M10)
- Osteoarthritis (M15-M19)
- Other joint disorders (M20-M25)

Systemic Connective Tissue Disorders (M30-M36)

Including:

- Systemic lupus erythematosus (M32)
- Dermatopolymyositis (M33)
- Systemic sclerosis (M34)
- Sjögren syndrome (M35.0)
- Other connective tissue disorders (M35)

Dorsopathies (M40-M54)

Spine conditions:

- Kyphosis/lordosis (M40)
- Scoliosis (M41)
- Spinal stenosis (M48)
- Intervertebral disc disorders (M50-M51)
- Low back pain (M54.5)
- Cervicalgia (M54.2)

Soft Tissue Disorders (M60-M79)

Categories include:

- Myositis (M60)
- Synovitis/tenosynovitis (M65)
- Rotator cuff disorders (M75)
- Enthesopathies (M76-M77)

- Fibromyalgia (M79.7)

Bone Disorders (M80-M90)

Covering:

- Osteoporosis (M80-M81)
- Osteomyelitis (M86)
- Osteonecrosis (M87)
- Paget's disease (M88)
- Complex regional pain syndrome (M89.0)

Coding guidelines:

Site Specification:

- Laterality
- Anatomical location
- Joint involvement
- Bone segment

Documentation Requirements:

- Acuity
- Cause/type
- Severity
- Associated manifestations
- Treatment status

Multiple Code Scenarios:

- Underlying conditions
- Manifestations
- Complications
- Pain syndromes

Key Indicators:

- Traumatic vs pathological
- Initial vs subsequent
- Acute vs chronic
- Disease stage

Clinical Documentation Needs:

- Imaging findings
- Physical exam results
- Functional status
- Treatment response

Specific Attention to:

- Pain location/severity
- Range of motion
- Weight-bearing status
- Functional limitations

Remember to Include:

- Injury type if applicable
- Healing status
- Surgical status
- Fracture type/pattern

GENITOURINARY SYSTEM

Kidney disorders (N00-N19)

Including:

- Glomerular diseases (N00-N08)
- Acute nephritis (N10)
- Chronic kidney disease (N18)
- Renal failure (N17-N19)
- Kidney stones (N20)
- Renal tubular disorders (N25)

Urinary system (N30-N39)

Conditions covering:

- Cystitis (N30)
- Bladder disorders (N31-N32)
- Urethritis (N34)
- Urethral stricture (N35)

- Urinary incontinence (N39.3-N39.4)
- UTI (N39.0)

Male genital disorders (N40-N51)

Including:

- Prostatic hyperplasia (N40)
- Prostatitis (N41)
- Hydrocele/spermatocele (N43)
- Orchitis/epididymitis (N45)
- Male infertility (N46)
- Erectile dysfunction (N52)

Female genital disorders (N60-N98)

Covering:

- Breast disorders (N60-N64)
- Inflammatory disorders (N70-N77)
- Endometriosis (N80)
- Prolapse (N81)
- Menstrual disorders (N91-N92)
- Female infertility (N97)

Coding guidelines:

Documentation Requirements:

- Acuity (acute/chronic)
- Stage/severity
- Causative factors
- Associated conditions
- Treatment status

Key Components:

- Location specificity
- Type of disorder
- Manifestations
- Complications
- Treatment response

Multiple Code Situations:

- Underlying conditions
- Manifestations
- Complications
- Associated symptoms

Special Considerations:

- CKD staging
- Dialysis status
- Transplant status
- Infection specifics

Clinical Indicators Needed:

- Laboratory values
- Imaging results
- Procedure findings
- Treatment outcomes

Remember to Document:

- Disease progression
- Complication presence
- Risk factors
- Associated conditions

Important Specifications:

- Laterality when applicable
- Infection type/organism
- Acute vs chronic status
- Treatment phase

Attention Required for:

- Staging documentation
- Causal relationships
- Treatment compliance
- Outcome measures

PREGNANCY AND CHILDBIRTH

Pregnancy with abortive outcome (O00-O08)

Including:

- Ectopic pregnancy (O00)
- Hydatidiform mole (O01)
- Other abnormal products (O02)
- Spontaneous abortion (O03)
- Medical abortion (O04)
- Complications following abortion (O08)

Antenatal care/complications (O09-O48)

Major categories:

- High-risk pregnancy (O09)
- Hemorrhage (O20, O46)
- Hypertensive disorders (O10-O16)
- Gestational diabetes (O24)
- Multiple gestation (O30-O31)
- Maternal care related to fetus (O32-O36)
- Preterm labor (O60.0)

Labor and delivery (O60-O77)

Covering:

- Preterm/term labor (O60)
- Failed induction (O61)
- Abnormal labor (O62)
- Long/obstructed labor (O63-O64)
- Umbilical complications (O69)
- Perineal lacerations (O70)

Complications of puerperium (O85-O92)

Including:

- Puerperal sepsis (O85)
- Venous complications (O87)

- Obstetric embolism (O88)
- Mental disorders (O90.6)
- Mastitis (O91)
- Lactation disorders (O92)

Coding guidelines:

Trimester Specification Required:

- First (less than 14 weeks)
- Second (14-28 weeks)
- Third (28 weeks until delivery)

Documentation Requirements:

- Gestational age
- Episode of care
- Outcome of delivery
- Complications
- Status of mother/fetus

Sequencing Rules:

- Principal diagnosis
- Outcome of delivery
- Complications
- Concurrent conditions

Additional Code Requirements:

- Supervision codes
- Fetal conditions
- Underlying conditions
- Social factors

Key Documentation Elements:

- Weeks of gestation
- Delivery method
- Multiple gestation status
- Previous cesarean status

Remember to Include:

- Maternal conditions

- Fetal conditions
- Placental conditions
- Amniotic fluid status

Special Attention to:

- Pre-existing conditions
- Pregnancy-induced conditions
- Complications
- Delivery outcome

Important Indicators:

- Risk factors
- Complications
- Treatment responses
- Monitoring needs

Code Requirements:

- Z3A code for weeks of gestation
- Delivery outcome when applicable
- Multiple gestation status
- Supervision requirements

SKIN CONDITIONS

Infections of skin (L00-L08)

Including:

- Staphylococcal scalded skin syndrome (L00)
- Impetigo (L01)
- Cutaneous abscess/furuncle (L02)
- Cellulitis (L03)
- Acute lymphadenitis (L04)
- Pilonidal cyst (L05)

Bullous disorders (L10-L14)

Covering:

- Pemphigus (L10)
- Pemphigoid (L12)
- Dermatitis herpetiformis (L13)
- Other bullous disorders (L14)

Dermatitis and eczema (L20-L30)

Including:

- Atopic dermatitis (L20)
- Seborrheic dermatitis (L21)
- Contact dermatitis (L23-L25)
- Nummular dermatitis (L30.0)
- Dyshidrosis (L30.1)

Papulosquamous disorders (L40-L45)

Categories:

- Psoriasis (L40)
- Parapsoriasis (L41)
- Pityriasis rosea (L42)
- Lichen planus (L43)
- Other papulosquamous disorders (L44)

Urticaria and erythema (L50-L54)

Including:

- Urticaria (L50)
- Erythema multiforme (L51)
- Erythema nodosum (L52)
- Toxic erythema (L53)

Disorders of skin appendages (L60-L75)

Covering:

- Nail disorders (L60)

- Hair disorders (L63-L66)
- Follicular disorders (L70-L73)
- Eccrine/apocrine disorders (L74-L75)

Coding guidelines:

Documentation Requirements:

- Location/distribution
- Acuity (acute/chronic)
- Severity
- Causative factors
- Associated symptoms

Key Components:

- Type of lesion
- Pattern/distribution
- Associated conditions
- Treatment response
- Complications

Important Specifications:

- Underlying causes
- Contributing factors
- Environmental triggers
- Treatment history

Clinical Indicators:

- Lesion characteristics
- Distribution pattern
- Associated symptoms
- Systemic involvement

Remember to Document:

- Lesion appearance
- Size/extent
- Duration
- Previous treatments
- Aggravating factors

Special Attention to:

- Infection status
- Allergic components
- Systemic conditions
- Environmental factors

Clinical Assessment Needs:

- Visual examination
- Culture results if applicable
- Biopsy findings
- Treatment response

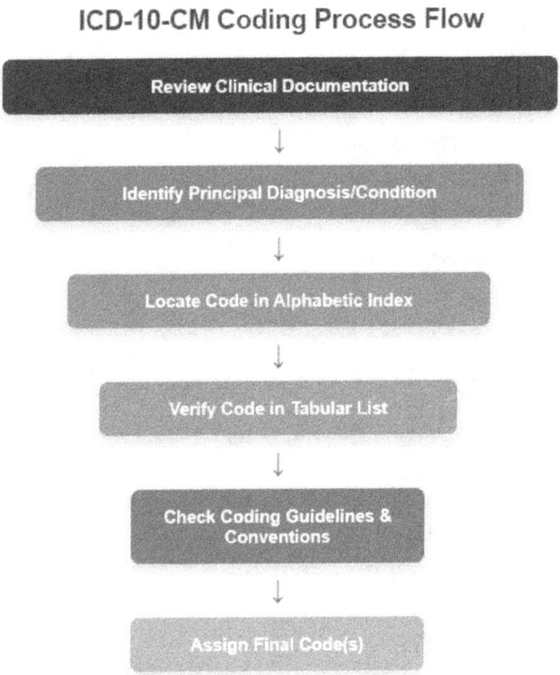

Summary

Medical coding using ICD-10-CM requires comprehensive understanding of disease processes, anatomical systems, and coding guidelines. The classification system provides detailed categorization across major body systems from infectious diseases to skin conditions. Each category demands specific documentation elements including disease type, acuity, severity, manifestations, and treatment status. Accurate code assignment depends on proper documentation of anatomical locations, causative factors, complications, and clinical indicators. Understanding combination codes, sequencing rules, and multiple code requirements ensures complete diagnostic representation. Proper documentation must include relevant clinical findings, laboratory results, imaging studies, and treatment responses to support code selection. The system emphasizes precision in identifying disease processes while maintaining standardized coding practices across healthcare settings.

Multiple Choice Questions

1. Which code range covers intestinal infections in ICD-10-CM?
   a) A15-A19
   b) A00-A09
   c) A20-A49
   d) B00-B34

2. Tuberculosis affecting other body systems is coded under:
   a) A15
   b) A18

c) A19
d) A16

3. The code range B00-B34 encompasses:
   a) Bacterial diseases
   b) Parasitic diseases
   c) Viral infections
   d) Mycoses

4. Secondary malignancies of lymph nodes are coded under:
   a) C77
   b) C78
   c) C79
   d) C80

5. Type 2 diabetes mellitus is coded under:
   a) E08
   b) E10
   c) E11
   d) E13

6. Which category includes substance-related disorders?
   a) F01-F09
   b) F10-F19
   c) F20-F29
   d) F30-F39

7. Hypertensive heart and kidney disease is coded under:
   a) I10
   b) I11

c) I12
d) I13

8. Acute nasopharyngitis is coded under:
   a) J00
   b) J01
   c) J02
   d) J03

9. GERD is classified under code:
   a) K20
   b) K21
   c) K22
   d) K23

10. Rheumatoid arthritis falls under code range:
    a) M00-M02
    b) M05-M06
    c) M10-M14
    d) M15-M19

11. Chronic kidney disease is coded under:
    a) N17
    b) N18
    c) N19
    d) N20

12. Ectopic pregnancy is coded under:
    a) O00
    b) O01
    c) O02
    d) O03

13. Which code range includes bullous disorders of skin?

a) L00-L08
b) L10-L14
c) L20-L30
d) L40-L45

14. Sepsis is coded under range:
    a) A20-A28
    b) A30-A39
    c) A40-A41
    d) A50-A64

15. Multiple sclerosis is coded under:
    a) G30
    b) G35
    c) G40
    d) G45

16. Status asthmaticus is coded under:
    a) J45
    b) J46
    c) J47
    d) J48

17. Acute pancreatitis is classified under:
    a) K85
    b) K86
    c) K87
    d) K88

18. Systemic lupus erythematosus is coded under:
    a) M30
    b) M31
    c) M32
    d) M33

19. Female infertility is coded under:
    a) N95
    b) N96
    c) N97
    d) N98

20. Contact dermatitis falls under code range:
    a) L20-L22
    b) L23-L25
    c) L26-L28
    d) L30-L32

21. Bacterial meningitis is coded under:
    a) G00
    b) G01
    c) G02
    d) G03

22. Malignant neoplasms of breast are coded under:
    a) C45
    b) C48
    c) C50
    d) C55

23. Which code range includes disorders of thyroid gland?
    a) E00-E07
    b) E10-E14
    c) E15-E19
    d) E20-E35

24. Acute myocardial infarction is coded under:
    a) I20
    b) I21

c) I22
d) I23

25. Cellulitis is coded under:
a) L00
b) L01
c) L02
d) L03

List of Important Questions

1. Explain the major differences between coding infectious diseases and neoplasms in ICD-10-CM.
2. How does ICD-10-CM classify diabetes mellitus, and what documentation elements are essential?
3. Discuss the coding guidelines for hypertensive diseases with multiple system involvement.
4. What are the key considerations when coding mental health conditions with substance use disorders?
5. Explain the documentation requirements for coding neoplasms with metastasis.
6. How are respiratory conditions coded when multiple sites are involved?
7. Describe the coding process for complex endocrine disorders with multiple manifestations.
8. What documentation elements are crucial for coding pregnancy complications?
9. How does ICD-10-CM handle coding for chronic conditions with acute exacerbations?
10. Explain the coding guidelines for musculoskeletal conditions with multiple site involvement.
11. What are the essential elements for coding digestive system disorders with complications?
12. How are skin conditions coded when multiple manifestations are present?
13. Discuss the coding requirements for nervous system disorders with multiple manifestations.
14. What are the key considerations when coding genitourinary conditions?
15. How does ICD-10-CM handle coding for post-procedural complications?
16. Explain the documentation requirements for coding circulatory system disorders.
17. What are the essential elements for coding infectious diseases with drug resistance?

18. How are mental health conditions coded when multiple diagnoses are present?
19. Discuss the coding guidelines for endocrine disorders with systemic manifestations.
20. What documentation is required for coding neoplasms with associated conditions??

Bibliography

1. Bowman SE. Health Information Management. 5th ed. Chicago: AHIMA Press; 2023.
2. Buck CJ. Step-by-Step Medical Coding 2024 Edition. Philadelphia: Elsevier; 2023.
3. Safian SC. ICD-10-CM Diagnostic Coding System: Education, Planning and Implementation. Burlington: Jones & Bartlett Learning; 2022.
4. O'Heron CT, Jarvis WR. ICD-10-CM Expert 2024. Salt Lake City: Optum360; 2023.
5. Schmidt M, Schmidt SAJ, Sandegaard JL, et al. The Danish National Patient Registry: a review of content, data quality, and research potential. Clin Epidemiol. 2015;7:449-490.
6. Quan H, Sundararajan V, Halfon P, et al. Coding algorithms for defining comorbidities in ICD-9-CM and ICD-10 administrative data. Med Care. 2005;43(11):1130-1139.
7. Southern DA, Pincus HA, Romano PS, et al. Enhanced capture of healthcare-related harms and injuries in the 11th revision of the International Classification of Diseases (ICD-11). Int J Qual Health Care. 2016;28(1):136-142.
8. Centers for Medicare & Medicaid Services. ICD-10-CM Official Guidelines for Coding and Reporting FY 2024. Baltimore: CMS; 2023.
9. World Health Organization. International Statistical Classification of Diseases and Related Health Problems, 10th Revision (ICD-10). Geneva: WHO; 2019.
10. Utter GH, Cox GL, Owens PL, Romano PS. Challenges and opportunities with ICD-10-CM/PCS: implications for surgical research involving administrative data. J Am Coll Surg. 2013;217(3):516-526.
11. O'Malley KJ, Cook KF, Price MD, et al. Measuring

diagnoses: ICD code accuracy. Health Serv Res. 2005;40(5):1620-1639.

12. Romano PS, Mark DH. Bias in the coding of hospital discharge data and its implications for quality assessment. Med Care. 1994;32(1):81-90.
13. Injury Surveillance Workgroup. Consensus Recommendations for Using Hospital Discharge Data for Injury Surveillance. Marietta: State and Territorial Injury Prevention Directors Association; 2003.
14. Stein HD, Nadkarni P, Erdos J, Miller PL. Exploring the degree of concordance of coded and textual data in answering clinical queries from a clinical data repository. J Am Med Inform Assoc. 2000;7(1):42-54.
15. Burns EM, Rigby E, Mamidanna R, et al. Systematic review of discharge coding accuracy. J Public Health (Oxf). 2012;34(1):138-148.
16. Campbell SE, Campbell MK, Grimshaw JM, Walker AE. A systematic review of discharge coding accuracy. J Public Health Med. 2001;23(3):205-211.
17. Hsia DC, Krushat WM, Fagan AB, et al. Accuracy of diagnostic coding for Medicare patients under the prospective-payment system. N Engl J Med. 1988;318(6):352-355.
18. Romano PS, Roos LL, Jollis JG. Adapting a clinical comorbidity index for use with ICD-9-CM administrative data: differing perspectives. J Clin Epidemiol. 1993;46(10):1075-1079.
19. Leibson CL, Needleman J, Buerhaus P, et al. Identifying in-hospital venous thromboembolism (VTE): a comparison of claims-based approaches with the Rochester Epidemiology Project VTE cohort. Med Care. 2008;46(2):127-132.
20. Drösler SE, Romano PS, Tancredi DJ, Klazinga NS.

International comparability of patient safety indicators in 15 OECD member countries: a methodological approach of adjustment by secondary diagnoses. Health Serv Res. 2012;47(1):275-292.

CHAPTER 7

INJURY AND EXTERNAL CAUSE CODING

Author

Dr Raghu Ram Jampala, Professor, Department of Pharmacy Practice, Sultan-ul-Uloom College of Pharmacy, Hyderabad, Telangana, India

Abstract

Trauma and injury coding in ICD-10-CM encompasses a comprehensive classification system for documenting various types of injuries, their causes, and outcomes. The coding structure follows anatomical organization, beginning with head and neck injuries (S00-S19), proceeding through thorax and trunk (S20-S39), to extremities (S40-S99). Effects and complications codes (T07-T88) cover multiple body regions, foreign bodies, burns, frostbite, poisoning, and various complications. External cause codes document the circumstances of injuries, including transport accidents (V00-V99), falls, exposure to forces, and intentional harm. The system incorporates place of occurrence (Y92) and activity codes (Y93) to provide context. Encounter classification uses 7th character extensions to distinguish between initial (A) and subsequent encounters (D), with specific indicators for healing status. Sequela coding (S) documents late effects of injuries, requiring clear documentation of the time gap between original injury and resulting condition. Multiple injury coding follows a hierarchy prioritizing the most severe injuries, with specific guidelines for combining injuries and sequencing codes. This structured approach ensures accurate documentation of injury severity, causation, treatment phase, and outcomes in medical records.

Keywords: *Injury classification; External cause codes; Encounter designation; Sequela documentation; Multiple trauma coding*

Learning Objectives

After completion of the chapter, the learners should be able to:

- Differentiate between anatomical injury codes and identify appropriate code ranges for specific body regions.
- Apply external cause codes correctly to document injury circumstances, including transport accidents and environmental exposures.
- Demonstrate proper use of 7th character extensions for initial encounters, subsequent visits, and sequela documentation.
- Select appropriate Y92 and Y93 codes to indicate place of occurrence and activity during injury.
- Apply multiple injury coding guidelines, including proper sequencing of primary and secondary injuries.
- Identify and document healing status variations and complications in injury recovery using appropriate modifiers

TRAUMA AND INJURY CODING

Head/Neck (S00-S19)

- Head injuries (S00-S09)
- Neck injuries (S10-S19)

Thorax/Trunk (S20-S39)

- Thorax injuries (S20-S29)
- Abdomen/lower back/pelvis (S30-S39)

Extremities (S40-S99)

Upper limb (S40-S69)

- Shoulder/upper arm (S40-S49)
- Elbow/forearm (S50-S59)
- Wrist/hand (S60-S69)

Lower limb (S70-S99)

- Hip/thigh (S70-S79)
- Knee/lower leg (S80-S89)
- Ankle/foot (S90-S99)

Effects/Complications (T07-T88)

- Multiple body regions (T07)
- Foreign bodies (T15-T19)
- Burns/corrosions (T20-T32)
- Frostbite (T33-T34)
- Poisoning (T36-T50)
- Toxic effects (T51-T65)
- Other external effects (T66-T78)
- Complications (T80-T88)

EXTERNAL CAUSE CODES

Transport Accidents (V00-V99)

- Pedestrian (V00-V09)
- Pedal cyclist (V10-V19)
- Motorcycle rider (V20-V29)
- Vehicle occupant (V30-V79)
- Other land transport (V80-V89)
- Water/air transport (V90-V99)

Other External **Causes (W00-X58)**

- Falls (W00-W19)
- Exposure to forces (W20-W49)
- Accidental drowning (W65-W74)

- Other accidental threats to breathing (W75-W84)
- Electric current/radiation (W85-W99)
- Fire/heat/hot substances (X00-X19)
- Natural forces (X30-X39)
- Poisoning/exposure (X40-X58)

Intent Codes (X71-Y09)

- Self-harm (X71-X83)
- Assault (X92-Y09)

Place of Occurrence (Y92)

- Home (Y92.0)
- Residential institution (Y92.1)
- School (Y92.2)
- Sports area (Y92.3)
- Street/highway (Y92.4)
- Public area (Y92.5)

Activity Codes (Y93)

- Sports activities (Y93.0)
- Leisure activities (Y93.1)
- Working (Y93.2)
- Educational (Y93.3)

Table. Common External Cause Scenarios and Their Code Assignments

Scenario Type	Code Range	Required Elements	Additional Coding
Transport Accidents	V00-V99	Vehicle type, Role of patient, Circumstances	Place of occurrence
Falls	W00-W19	Height, Surface type, Circumstance	Activity code
Sports Injuries	Y93.0	Specific sport, Location	Type of injury

Scenario Type	Code Range	Required Elements	Additional Coding
Occupational	Y93.2	Work environment, Activity	Nature of injury
Assault	X92-Y09	Method, Intent	Place code
Environmental	X30-X39	Nature of exposure	Activity code

INITIAL VS. SUBSEQUENT ENCOUNTERS

7th character extensions

Initial Encounter (A)

- Emergency encounter
- Initial evaluation
- Active treatment
- Surgical treatment

Subsequent Encounter (D)

- Routine healing (D1)
- Delayed healing (D2)
- Problem healing (D3)
- Aftercare visits
- Follow-up care

Medical Care Status

- Routine healing
- Delayed healing
- Nonunion
- Malunion
- Complications

Table. Seventh Character Extensions and Their Applications in Injury Coding

Extension	Description	Common Scenarios	Documentation Requirements
A (Initial)	Active treatment phase	Emergency visits, First evaluation, Surgical treatment	Acute injury details, Treatment plan
D1	Routine healing	Normal follow-up care	Progress notes, Expected healing
D2	Delayed healing	Slower than expected	Healing complications, Intervention plans
D3	Problem healing	Complications present	Specific complications, Modified treatment
S (Sequela)	Late effects	Residual conditions	Original injury link, Time gap

SEQUELA

Late effects of injuries (T90-T98)

- Brain injury (T90.5)
- Spinal cord injury (T91.3)
- Fractures (T90.2, T91.2, T92.2, T93.2)
- Burns (T95)
- Poisoning (T96)
- Other trauma (T98)

Sequela Coding Rules:

- Use (S) as 7th character
- Code both sequela and original injury

- Link current condition to original injury
- Time gap must be documented

MULTIPLE INJURY CODING

Hierarchy Guidelines

Most Severe Injury First

- Life-threatening conditions
- Highest mortality risk
- Greatest resource use

Injury Combinations

- Head injuries with other sites (S00-S09)
- Spinal injuries with fractures (S12-S32)
- Multiple fractures (T02)
- Multiple wounds (T01)
- Multiple burns (T29)

Coding Order

- Principal injury (most severe)
- Additional injuries (anatomic order)
- Associated complications
- External cause codes

Special Circumstances

- Bilateral injuries
- Multiple sites same type
- Combined injuries
- Crush injuries (T04)

Table. Multiple Injury Priority Coding Guidelines

Priority Level	Injury Type	Examples	Coding Notes
Level 1	Life-threatening	Intracranial injury, Major vessel injury	Code first
Level 2	Major trauma	Multiple fractures, Crush injuries	Code after life-threatening
Level 3	Significant soft tissue	Deep wounds, Burns	Code in anatomical order
Level 4	Minor injuries	Superficial injuries, Contusions	Code last
Special Cases	Bilateral/Multiple sites	Same injury type on multiple sites	Use combination codes

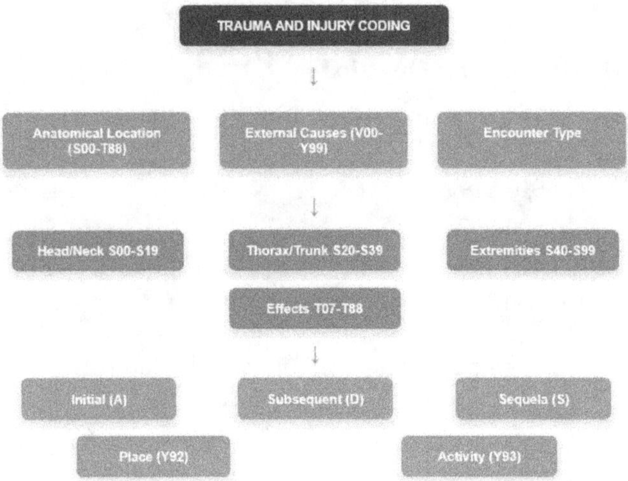

Summary

Medical coding for trauma and injuries follows a systematic organization within ICD-10-CM, utilizing S00-T88 codes for anatomical classifications and specific injury types. The system progresses from head injuries through extremities while incorporating effects and complications. External cause codes (V00-X58) document the circumstances surrounding injuries, including transport accidents, falls, and intentional harm. Additional codes capture the place of occurrence (Y92) and activity during injury (Y93). Critical distinctions between initial and subsequent encounters are made through 7th character extensions, with specific designations for healing status. Sequela coding addresses late effects of injuries, requiring proper documentation and linkage to original injuries. Multiple injury situations follow a structured hierarchy, prioritizing life-threatening conditions and following specific guidelines for injury combinations and coding sequence.

Multiple Choice Questions

1. Which code range represents head injuries in ICD-10-CM?
   a) S10-S19
   b) S00-S09
   c) S20-S29
   d) S30-S39

2. The 7th character 'A' in injury codes indicates:
   a) Subsequent encounter
   b) Initial encounter

c) Sequela
d) Routine healing

3. Transport accidents involving pedestrians are coded using:
   a) V00-V09
   b) V10-V19
   c) V20-V29
   d) V30-V79

4. Burns and corrosions are classified under:
   a) T15-T19
   b) T33-T34
   c) T20-T32
   d) T36-T50

5. Which Y92 code represents injuries occurring in school?
   a) Y92.0
   b) Y92.1
   c) Y92.2
   d) Y92.5

6. Late effects of brain injury are coded using:
   a) T90.2
   b) T90.5
   c) T91.3
   d) T95

7. For subsequent encounters with delayed healing, which 7th character is used?
   a) D1
   b) D2

c) D3
d) S

8. Multiple body regions injuries are coded under:
   a) T01
   b) T02
   c) T07
   d) T29

9. Activity codes for sports activities fall under:
   a) Y93.0
   b) Y93.1
   c) Y93.2
   d) Y93.3

10. Which code range represents lower limb injuries?
    a) S40-S69
    b) S60-S69
    c) S70-S99
    d) S90-S99

11. Foreign body codes are found in range:
    a) T07-T14
    b) T15-T19
    c) T20-T32
    d) T33-T34

12. Self-harm codes are classified under:
    a) X71-X83
    b) X92-Y09
    c) Y92
    d) Y93

13. The code range for motorcycle rider accidents is:
    a) V00-V09

b) V10-V19
c) V20-V29
d) V30-V79

14. Problems with healing in subsequent encounters use 7th character:
a) A
b) D1
c) D2
d) D3

15. Spinal cord injury sequela is coded as:
a) T90.5
b) T91.2
c) T91.3
d) T92.2

16. The code range for exposure to forces is:
a) W00-W19
b) W20-W49
c) W65-W74
d) W85-W99

17. Which represents the correct coding order for multiple injuries?
a) External cause first
b) Most severe injury first
c) Anatomical order
d) Chronological order

18. Poisoning and toxic effects are coded in range:
a) T36-T50
b) T51-T65

c) Both a and b
d) T66-T78

19. Residential institution injuries are coded under:
a) Y92.0
b) Y92.1
c) Y92.2
d) Y92.3

20. The code range for wrist and hand injuries is:
a) S40-S49
b) S50-S59
c) S60-S69
d) S70-S79

21. Educational activities are coded under:
a) Y93.0
b) Y93.1
c) Y93.2
d) Y93.3

22. Multiple fractures are coded under:
a) T01
b) T02
c) T04
d) T07

23. For sequela coding, which must be documented?
a) Original injury
b) Current condition
c) Time gap
d) All of the above

24. Assault codes fall under:
a) X71-X83

b) X92-Y09
c) Y92
d) W85-W99

25. The code range for water and air transport accidents is:
a) V30-V79
b) V80-V89
c) V90-V99
d) W00-W19

List of Important Questions

1. Explain the hierarchical approach to coding multiple injuries and discuss its significance in medical coding.
2. How do 7th character extensions differentiate between initial and subsequent encounters? Provide examples.
3. Describe the process of coding sequela injuries and explain the documentation requirements.
4. Compare and contrast the coding requirements for upper and lower extremity injuries.
5. What are the key considerations when coding transport accidents? Discuss the different categories.
6. Explain the importance of external cause codes in injury coding and their proper application.
7. How are burns and corrosions coded in ICD-10-CM? Discuss the factors affecting code selection.
8. Describe the proper coding sequence for multiple trauma cases involving head injuries.
9. What role do place of occurrence and activity codes play in injury coding?
10. Discuss the coding guidelines for poisoning and toxic effects.
11. How are complications of trauma coded? Provide examples.
12. Explain the difference between routine, delayed, and problem healing in subsequent encounters.
13. What are the special considerations when coding bilateral injuries?
14. Describe the coding process for crush injuries and multiple site injuries.
15. How are self-harm and assault injuries distinguished in coding?
16. Discuss the importance of proper documentation in trauma coding.

17. What are the key elements in coding foreign body injuries?
18. Explain the coding guidelines for frostbite injuries.
19. How are late effects of injuries coded and documented?
20. Discuss the role of anatomical specificity in injury coding?

Bibliography

1. Netter JZ, Smith MA. ICD-10-CM Expert for Physicians 2024. Chicago: American Medical Association; 2023.
2. Butler KH, Marx J, Bounds R. Rosen's Emergency Medicine: Concepts and Clinical Practice. 10th ed. Philadelphia: Elsevier; 2023.
3. Abraham M, Ahlman JT, Boudreau AJ, Connelly JL. CPT 2024 Professional Edition. Chicago: American Medical Association; 2023.
4. Benson M, Fixsen R, Macleod M. Essential ICD-10 Coding Handbook. Health Administration Press; 2022.
5. Schmidt TA, Cone DC. Emergency Medical Services: Clinical Practice and Systems Oversight. 3rd ed. Wiley-Blackwell; 2021.
6. Buck CJ. Step-by-Step Medical Coding. 2024 Edition. St. Louis: Elsevier; 2023.
7. Safian SC, Johnson-Carlson P. Health Information Management Technology: An Applied Approach. 6th ed. AHIMA Press; 2020.
8. Leon-Chisen N. ICD-10-PCS Code Book, 2024. Chicago: American Hospital Association; 2023.
9. Judd KS, Pack RE. Clinical Documentation Improvement: Principles and Practice. AHIMA Press; 2020.
10. O'Sullivan SB, Schmitz TJ, Fulk G. Physical Rehabilitation. 7th ed. Philadelphia: F.A. Davis Company; 2019.
11. Proctor ML, Adams JG. Emergency Medicine: Clinical Essentials. 3rd ed. Philadelphia: Elsevier; 2022.
12. Anderson KN. Mosby's Medical Dictionary. 10th ed. St. Louis: Elsevier; 2021.
13. Nichols A. Coding With Modifiers: A Guide to Correct CPT and HCPCS Level II Modifier Usage.

American Medical Association; 2023.

14. Slee VN, Slee DA, Schmidt HJ. Health Care Terms. 6th ed. Tringa Press; 2021.
15. Anwar R, Li L. Medical Coding Study Guide. J Am Health Inf Manag Assoc. 2022;93(4):24-31.
16. Johnson KA, Sympson S. ICD-10-CM and ICD-10-PCS Coding Handbook 2024. Chicago: American Hospital Association; 2023.
17. Dorland WA. Dorland's Illustrated Medical Dictionary. 34th ed. Philadelphia: Elsevier; 2020.
18. Hapuarachchi T, Smith M. Understanding Medical Coding: A Comprehensive Guide. J Med Syst. 2021;45(3):1-12.
19. Green MA, Rowell JC. Understanding Health Insurance: A Guide to Billing and Reimbursement. 15th ed. Cengage Learning; 2023.
20. Roberts D, Heinrich N. Medical Coding Quality Review: Guidelines and Best Practices. Health Inf Manage J. 2022;51(2):89-97.

CHAPTER 8

SIGNS, SYMPTOMS, AND ILL-DEFINED CONDITIONS

Author

Miss Kumari Preeti, Assistant Professor, Vidyawati Devi College of Pharmacy, Salempur, Deoria, Uttar Pradesh, India

Abstract

The classification and usage of R-codes (R00-R99) encompasses signs, symptoms, and ill-defined conditions in healthcare settings. A systematic categorization of symptoms spans major body systems including circulatory, respiratory, digestive, skin, nervous, musculoskeletal, and urinary systems, along with cognitive and general symptoms. Clear guidelines establish when to code signs and symptoms as primary or secondary diagnoses, emphasizing their use when no definitive diagnosis exists or when symptoms require additional monitoring beyond the primary condition. Distinct differences exist between inpatient and outpatient coding practices for uncertain diagnoses, with inpatient settings allowing coding of probable, suspected, or rule-out conditions, while outpatient settings require coding only confirmed diagnoses or presenting symptoms. Documentation requirements include symptom description, duration, severity, and treatment provided. Handling rule-out conditions and unspecified codes requires careful attention to documentation accuracy and appropriate use when clinical information is limited or unavailable.

Keywords: *R-codes; symptom classification; diagnostic uncertainty; documentation requirements; coding guidelines*

Learning Objectives

After completion of the chapter, the learner should be able to:

- Identify and classify R-codes according to body systems and symptom categories
- Differentiate between appropriate uses of signs and symptoms as primary versus secondary diagnoses
- Apply correct coding guidelines for uncertain diagnoses in both inpatient and outpatient settings
- Evaluate documentation requirements for proper assignment of symptom codes
- Demonstrate proper usage of unspecified codes and understanding of rule-out conditions
- Recognize when to query healthcare providers for additional documentation clarity.

R CODES USAGE

Symptoms/Signs Involving:

Circulatory/Respiratory (R00-R09)

- Heart rhythms/beats (R00)
- Blood pressure (R03)
- Breathing abnormalities (R06)
- Chest pain (R07)
- Hemorrhage (R04)

Digestive/Abdomen (R10-R19)

- Abdominal pain (R10)
- Nausea/vomiting (R11)
- Diarrhea (R15)

- Jaundice (R17)
- Ascites (R18)

Skin/Subcutaneous (R20-R23)

- Sensory disturbances (R20)
- Rash (R21)
- Skin changes (R23)

Nervous/Musculoskeletal (R25-R29)

- Abnormal movements (R25)
- Gait abnormalities (R26)
- Coordination issues (R27)
- Reflexes (R29)

Urinary System (R30-R39)

- Urinary frequency (R35)
- Retention (R33)
- Stream abnormalities (R39)

Cognition/Perception/Emotion (R40-R46)

- Somnolence/stupor/coma (R40)
- Cognitive deficits (R41)
- Dizziness (R42)
- Speech disturbances (R47)

General Symptoms (R50-R69)

- Fever (R50)
- Headache (R51)
- Pain, general (R52)
- Malaise/fatigue (R53)
- Convulsions (R56)

Table. Common Signs and Symptoms by Body System with R-Codes

Body System	R-Code Range	Common Symptoms	Documentation Requirements
Circulatory/Respiratory	R00-R09	Tachycardia, Dyspnea, Chest pain	Frequency, Duration, Location
Digestive/Abdomen	R10-R19	Abdominal pain, Nausea, Jaundice	Severity, Pattern, Associated symptoms
Skin/Subcutaneous	R20-R23	Rash, Numbness, Color changes	Distribution, Appearance, Progression
Nervous/Musculoskeletal	R25-R29	Tremor, Ataxia, Weakness	Location, Intensity, Frequency
Urinary	R30-R39	Frequency, Retention, Dysuria	Volume, Pattern, Associated pain
Cognitive/Emotional	R40-R46	Confusion, Anxiety, Memory loss	Onset, Duration, Impact on function
General	R50-R69	Fever, Fatigue, Pain	Measurements, Duration, Pattern

WHEN TO CODE SIGNS AND SYMPTOMS

Primary Diagnosis Coding

- When no definitive diagnosis established
- Signs/symptoms not routinely integral to disease process
- Multiple signs/symptoms without definitive diagnosis
- When signs/symptoms are the focus of treatment

Secondary Diagnosis Coding

- Not routinely part of disease
- Requires additional monitoring
- Affects patient care
- Independent of primary condition

Do Not Code When:

- Signs/symptoms are integral part of diagnosed condition
- Routinely associated with disease process
- Signs/symptoms naturally progress to diagnosis
- Diagnostic workup clearly indicates condition

Documentation Requirements:

- Clear description of symptoms
- Duration and severity
- Treatment provided
- Diagnostic studies performed

Table. Coding Decision Matrix for Signs and Symptoms

Scenario	Inpatient Setting	Outpatient Setting	Documentation Needed
Definitive diagnosis established	Do not code symptoms	Do not code symptoms	Final diagnosis
Rule-out conditions	Code as if exists	Code symptoms only	Clinical indicators
Multiple symptoms, no diagnosis	Code all relevant symptoms	Code all relevant symptoms	Each symptom described
Symptoms requiring monitoring	Code as secondary	Code as secondary	Monitoring parameters
Integral to known condition	Do not code separately	Do not code separately	Relationship to condition
Focus of treatment	Code as primary	Code as primary	Treatment plan

UNCERTAIN DIAGNOSES

Inpatient Setting

- Code diagnoses documented as "probable"
- Code "suspected" conditions
- Code "likely" diagnoses
- Code "questionable" conditions
- Code "rule out" diagnoses

Outpatient Setting

- Do not code uncertain diagnoses
- Code signs/symptoms instead

- Code to highest degree of certainty
- Wait for definitive diagnosis

Documentation Guidelines:

- Provider must document uncertainty
- Terms indicating probability
- Linking conditions
- Clinical evidence support

Coding Rules:

- Code only documented conditions
- No assumptions allowed
- Query provider if unclear
- Follow coding guidelines for setting

Table. Documentation Requirements for Uncertain Diagnoses

Setting	Acceptable Terms	Required Documentation	Coding Action
Inpatient	Probable, Suspected, Likely, Questionable	Clinical evidence, Diagnostic plans, Provider statement	Code condition
	Rule-out, Working diagnosis	Testing ordered, Clinical indicators	Code condition
	Possible, Cannot exclude	Supporting documentation, Clinical correlation	Code condition
Outpatient	Suspected, Rule-out	Signs and symptoms, Testing plans	Code symptoms
	Probable, Likely	Clinical findings, Diagnostic results	Code symptoms
	Possible, Query	Presenting complaints, Examination findings	Code symptoms

RULE-OUT CONDITIONS

In medical coding, handling "rule-out" conditions varies significantly between inpatient and outpatient settings. For inpatient cases, coders should code diagnoses that are being ruled out as if the condition exists. This practice exists because inpatient admissions often involve extensive diagnostic workups where multiple conditions are being evaluated simultaneously.

For outpatient encounters, the approach is markedly different. Coders should not code rule-out conditions; instead, they should code the presenting signs and symptoms that led to the diagnostic investigation. This continues until a definitive diagnosis is established.

Documentation must include:

- A clear statement of conditions being ruled out
- Clinical indicators supporting the investigation
- Diagnostic testing plans
- Clear follow-up protocols

UNSPECIFIED CONDITIONS

Unspecified codes serve an important purpose in medical coding, though their use should be limited when possible. These codes become necessary when clinical documentation lacks the specificity needed for a more detailed code, or when information is genuinely unknown at the time of encounter.

Common scenarios requiring unspecified codes include:

1. Initial encounters before diagnostic testing is complete
2. Emergency situations where detailed information isn't immediately available
3. Cases where the exact cause or manifestation

cannot be determined

Quality Improvement Perspective:

Healthcare facilities should monitor the use of unspecified codes as they often indicate opportunities for documentation improvement. Regular analysis can reveal patterns where additional provider education or documentation tools might be beneficial.

When working with unspecified conditions, remember that coders cannot make assumptions to assign more specific codes - they must code strictly based on the documented information. If more specific information is needed and available, a provider query may be appropriate.

Summary

Signs, symptoms, and ill-defined conditions form a critical component of medical coding through R-codes (R00-R99). The systematic organization of symptoms across body systems provides a structured approach to documenting patient conditions when definitive diagnoses are not established. Primary and secondary diagnosis coding guidelines help determine when to code symptoms independently versus when they are integral to known conditions. The distinction between inpatient and outpatient coding for uncertain diagnoses remains fundamental, particularly in handling rule-out conditions and unspecified codes. Proper documentation, including symptom characteristics, treatment approaches, and diagnostic studies, ensures accurate code assignment and supports quality patient care. Understanding when to use unspecified codes and managing uncertain diagnoses requires careful attention to coding guidelines specific to each healthcare setting.

Multiple Choice Questions

1. Which code series is used for signs, symptoms, and ill-defined conditions?
   a) S codes
   b) R codes
   c) T codes
   d) Q codes

2. In outpatient settings, how should "rule-out" conditions be coded?
   a) Code the suspected condition
   b) Code the signs and symptoms
   c) Code as confirmed diagnosis
   d) Do not code at all

3. When can signs and symptoms be coded as primary diagnosis?
   a) When integral to disease process
   b) When no definitive diagnosis is established
   c) When routinely associated with condition
   d) When diagnosis is confirmed

4. In inpatient settings, which type of diagnosis should be coded?
   a) Only confirmed diagnoses
   b) Only chronic conditions
   c) Probable and suspected conditions
   d) Only acute conditions

5. Signs and symptoms should NOT be coded when:
   a) They are the focus of treatment
   b) They affect patient care

c) They are integral part of diagnosed condition
d) They require additional monitoring

6. What is required in documentation for signs and symptoms?
a) Only duration
b) Only treatment provided
c) Only severity
d) All of the above

7. R00-R09 codes are used for symptoms involving:
a) Digestive system
b) Circulatory and respiratory systems
c) Skin conditions
d) Urinary system

8. When coding unspecified conditions:
a) Coders can make assumptions
b) Only code based on documented information
c) Always query the provider
d) Use most specific code possible without documentation

9. For outpatient encounters with uncertain diagnoses:
a) Code the suspected condition
b) Code signs and symptoms
c) Code probable diagnosis
d) Code rule-out condition

10. R codes R20-R23 relate to:
a) Digestive symptoms
b) Skin and subcutaneous symptoms

c) Nervous system symptoms
d) Urinary symptoms

11. Which symptom category includes headache?
a) Nervous system symptoms
b) General symptoms
c) Cognitive symptoms
d) Pain-specific symptoms

12. Secondary diagnosis coding of symptoms is appropriate when:
a) Symptoms are routine part of disease
b) No treatment is provided
c) Additional monitoring is required
d) Diagnosis is confirmed

13. Quality improvement in coding unspecified conditions involves:
a) Using them whenever possible
b) Never using them
c) Monitoring their use for documentation improvement
d) Ignoring them completely

14. R40-R46 codes involve:
a) Skin symptoms
b) Digestive symptoms
c) Cognition/perception/emotion symptoms
d) Urinary symptoms

15. Documentation for rule-out conditions must include:
a) Only diagnostic testing plans
b) Only clinical indicators

c) Only follow-up protocols
d) All of the above

16. In inpatient settings, which term indicates uncertainty?
a) Confirmed
b) Established
c) Probable
d) Definitive

17. R codes R10-R19 primarily deal with:
a) Respiratory symptoms
b) Digestive and abdominal symptoms
c) Skin symptoms
d) Nervous system symptoms

18. When can coders make assumptions about unspecified conditions?
a) When documentation is unclear
b) When provider is unavailable
c) When condition is obvious
d) Never

19. Which symptoms are included in R25-R29?
a) Digestive symptoms
b) Nervous and musculoskeletal symptoms
c) Urinary symptoms
d) Skin symptoms

20. For inpatient coding, "rule-out" conditions are coded as:
a) Not coded
b) Existing conditions

c) Secondary diagnoses only
d) Signs and symptoms only

21. What is required when coding signs and symptoms?
a) Patient's age
b) Clear description
c) Family history
d) Social history

22. R30-R39 codes are associated with:
a) Respiratory system
b) Digestive system
c) Urinary system
d) Nervous system

23. When dealing with uncertain diagnoses in outpatient settings:
a) Code to highest degree of certainty
b) Code all possibilities
c) Code suspected conditions
d) Code rule-out conditions

24. General symptoms (R50-R69) include:
a) Only fever
b) Only headache
c) Only malaise
d) All of these

25. Documentation guidelines for uncertain diagnoses require:
a) Provider must document uncertainty
b) Patient must confirm symptoms
c) Family history must be present
d) Social history must be documented

List of Important Questions

1. Explain the structure and significance of R-codes in medical coding. How are they organized by body systems?
2. Compare and contrast the coding guidelines for uncertain diagnoses between inpatient and outpatient settings.
3. What are the key criteria for coding signs and symptoms as primary diagnoses? Provide examples.
4. Discuss the documentation requirements for coding signs and symptoms. Why is proper documentation crucial?
5. How should rule-out conditions be handled differently in inpatient versus outpatient settings?
6. Explain the appropriate use of unspecified codes and their role in medical coding.
7. What are the major categories of symptoms involving the circulatory and respiratory systems (R00-R09)?
8. Describe the circumstances under which signs and symptoms should not be coded.
9. How do documentation requirements differ for uncertain diagnoses versus confirmed diagnoses?
10. What role does quality improvement play in the management of unspecified codes?
11. Explain the coding guidelines for secondary diagnosis of signs and symptoms.
12. What are the key considerations when coding cognitive and perceptual symptoms (R40-R46)?
13. Describe the documentation requirements for rule-out conditions.
14. How should coders handle multiple signs and symptoms without a definitive diagnosis?
15. What are the essential elements of documentation for uncertain diagnoses?

16. Discuss the importance of provider queries in symptom coding.
17. Explain the relationship between signs/symptoms and their associated definitive diagnoses.
18. How do general symptoms (R50-R69) differ from system-specific symptoms?
19. What are the key considerations when coding digestive and abdominal symptoms (R10-R19)?
20. Discuss the role of clinical indicators in coding uncertain diagnoses

Bibliography

1. Buck CJ. Step-by-Step Medical Coding, 2023 Edition. St. Louis: Elsevier; 2022.
2. American Medical Association. ICD-10-CM 2023: The Complete Official Codebook. Chicago: AMA Press; 2022.
3. Abraham M, Ahlman JT, Boudreau AJ, Connelly JL. CPT 2023 Professional Edition. Chicago: American Medical Association; 2022.
4. Safian SC. Understanding ICD-10-CM and ICD-10-PCS: A Worktext. Burlington: Jones & Bartlett Learning; 2021.
5. Bowman S. ICD-10-CM Documentation 2023: Essential Charting Guidance. Chicago: AHIMA Press; 2022.
6. O'Hara KE, Reed PS. Medical Records and the Law. Burlington: Jones & Bartlett Learning; 2021.
7. Fordney MT. Insurance Handbook for the Medical Office. St. Louis: Elsevier; 2021.
8. Proctor SE, Young-Adams AP. Kinn's The Medical Assistant. St. Louis: Elsevier; 2023.
9. Johnson KA, Terrell S. Medical Coding and Billing Guidelines. J AHIMA. 2022;93(6):16-20.
10. Smith JT, Brown RD. Clinical Documentation Improvement. Health Inf Manage J. 2021;50(1):28-35.
11. Centers for Medicare & Medicaid Services. ICD-10-CM Official Guidelines for Coding and Reporting FY 2023. Baltimore: CMS; 2022.
12. World Health Organization. International Classification of Diseases, 11th Revision (ICD-11). Geneva: WHO; 2022.
13. Anderson P, Willis GB. Coding Clinic Guidance: A Systematic Review. J AHIMA. 2021;92(8):32-37.
14. Roberts RF, Innes KC, Walker SM. Introducing ICD-11: The Next Generation. Med J Aust.

2022;216(2):85-87.
15. Harris M, Taylor G. Medical Statistics Made Easy. London: Scion Publishing; 2021.
16. Nobleman C, Davis N. Documentation Requirements for Risk Adjustment. J AHIMA. 2022;93(1):22-26.
17. American Hospital Association. Coding Clinic for ICD-10-CM and ICD-10-PCS. Chicago: AHA; 2023.
18. Wilson L, Goulding R. Understanding Healthcare Coding. Health Inf Manage. 2021;45(2):89-95.
19. Peterson AM, Kelly WN. Managing Pharmacy Practice: Principles, Strategies, and Systems. Boca Raton: CRC Press; 2021.
20. Thompson EG, Black WC. Coding Guidelines Update: Clinical Documentation. J Healthcare Manage. 2022;67(3):215-222.

CHAPTER 9

Z CODES AND SPECIAL CIRCUMSTANCES

Author

Mrs. Vinny Therissa Mangam, Assistant Professor, Department of Pharmaceutical Analysis, Aditya College of Pharmacy, Aditya University, Surampalem, Andhra Pradesh, India

Abstract

Z codes serve as essential indicators for healthcare encounters unrelated to disease or injury, encompassing various aspects of health status and care delivery. These codes span multiple categories including general examinations, screenings, potential health hazards, reproductive health, social circumstances, and follow-up care. Screening codes specifically target asymptomatic testing for early disease detection, while observation codes address evaluated but ruled-out conditions. Personal history codes document resolved conditions that may influence current care, particularly in areas such as previous malignancies, various diseases, and medical treatments. Status codes indicate ongoing conditions or situations affecting healthcare, including artificial openings, device dependence, and organ transplant status. Follow-up care codes document post-treatment surveillance and aftercare needs. Each category has specific documentation requirements and coding guidelines for proper implementation. The coding system emphasizes the importance of accurate sequencing, proper documentation support, and clear distinction between active and historical conditions. These codes play a crucial role in comprehensive health records by capturing circumstances affecting patient care, supporting medical necessity, and guiding treatment decisions.

Keywords: *Healthcare encounters; Medical coding; Patient surveillance; Health status documentation; Clinical documentation improvement*

Learning Objectives

After completion of the chapter, the learner should be able to:

- Differentiate between the major categories of Z codes and their appropriate usage in healthcare documentation
- Apply proper coding guidelines for screening and observation encounters, understanding the key distinctions between these types of visits
- Evaluate and accurately document personal history codes, ensuring proper distinction between historical and active conditions
- Implement status codes correctly to reflect ongoing conditions and their impact on current patient care
- Demonstrate proper documentation and sequencing of follow-up care codes in relation to primary diagnoses
- Identify and avoid common coding errors in Z code application, ensuring compliance with documentation requirements

FACTORS INFLUENCING HEALTH STATUS

Purpose and Usage

Z codes represent reasons for healthcare encounters that are not related to disease or injury. These codes capture important health-related circumstances and factors that influence care delivery and outcomes.

Categories:

General Examinations and Screenings (Z00-Z13)

These codes describe routine health checks, administrative exams, and screening procedures.

Examples include:

- Annual physical examinations
- Pre-employment screenings
- Vision and hearing checkups
- Special screening for specific diseases

Table. Z Code Categories and Their Applications

Z Code Range	Category	Common Applications	Documentation Requirements
Z00-Z13	General Examinations	Annual physicals, Pre-employment screenings	Purpose of exam, Findings
Z20-Z29	Potential Health Hazards	Disease exposure, Immunizations	Nature of exposure, Preventive measures
Z30-Z39	Reproductive Health	Contraception, Pregnancy care	Treatment details, Outcome
Z55-Z65	Social Circumstances	Employment, Housing issues	Specific circumstances, Impact on health
Z40-Z54	Follow-up Care	Post-surgical care, Rehabilitation	Treatment history, Current care plan

Potential Health Hazards (Z20-Z29)

Used to document exposure risks and preventive measures:

- Contact with communicable diseases
- Immunization status
- Need for prophylactic measures
- Environmental hazard exposure

Reproductive Health (Z30-Z39)

Covers encounters related to reproduction and childbirth:

- Contraceptive management
- Pregnancy supervision
- Outcome of delivery
- Postpartum care

Social and Personal Circumstances (Z55-Z65)

Documents factors affecting health status:

- Employment concerns
- Educational difficulties
- Social environment problems
- Housing or economic issues
- Family circumstances

Follow-up Care (Z40-Z54)

Used for ongoing care after treatment:

- Post-surgical aftercare
- Medical device adjustment
- Rehabilitation care
- Convalescence

Coding Guidelines:

Z codes may be used as primary or secondary diagnoses. They should be specific to the encounter's purpose. Documentation must support their use. Some Z codes require additional diagnosis codes

Remember: Z codes provide valuable information about circumstances affecting patient care and are essential for comprehensive health records.

SCREENING AND OBSERVATION CODES

Screening Codes (Z11-Z13)

Screening codes represent the testing of asymptomatic individuals to detect early disease or risk factors. Understanding proper screening code usage is essential for accurate coding:

Definition:

A screening is a test for a disease or precursor when no signs, symptoms, or associated diagnosis exists. The key distinction is that the patient has no symptoms related to the condition being screened.

Proper Usage Guidelines:

1. The screening code should be primary when the screening is the primary reason for the visit
2. If a condition is discovered during screening, the condition becomes primary, and the screening code becomes secondary
3. Additional procedures or diagnostic codes may be required to completely describe the service

Example:

A patient comes in for routine mammogram screening (Z12.31). If breast cancer is detected, the cancer code becomes primary, and Z12.31 becomes secondary.

Observation Codes (Z03-Z04)

Observation codes are used when a patient is being evaluated for a suspected condition that is ruled out. These codes have specific guidelines:

When to Use:

- Patient has signs/symptoms that suggest a serious condition
- After medical evaluation, the suspected condition is ruled out
- No definitive diagnosis is established
- Patient doesn't require further treatment

Key Points for Observation:

1. Must be used only when no injury or cause is found
2. Cannot be used with codes describing signs or symptoms
3. Explains why patient required medical evaluation
4. Documents medical necessity for the encounter

Documentation Requirements:

- Clear documentation of suspected condition
- Evidence of medical evaluation
- Documentation that condition was ruled out
- Any follow-up instructions

Important Distinctions:

- Screening: Testing without symptoms
- Observation: Evaluation of symptoms/concerns that are ruled out
- Diagnostic: Evaluation leading to a diagnosis

Table. Screening vs. Observation Code Comparison

Feature	Screening Codes (Z11-Z13)	Observation Codes (Z03-Z04)
Patient Status	Asymptomatic	Has signs/symptoms
Purpose	Early detection	Rule out suspected condition
Primary Usage	Preventive care	Evaluation of concerns
Sequencing	Primary when screening is main reason	Primary when no other diagnosis
Documentation Needs	Screening type, Results	Suspected condition, Evaluation results
Additional Coding	Procedure codes may be needed	Cannot use with symptom codes

HISTORY CODES

Understanding Personal History Codes (Z85-Z92)

Personal history codes document significant past medical conditions that may influence current care but are no longer active. These codes provide crucial information for ongoing risk assessment and care planning.

Categories of History Codes:

1. Personal History of Malignant Neoplasms (Z85)
   - Used when cancer is fully treated and no longer exists
   - Indicates location of previous cancer
   - Helps track cancer surveillance needs
   - Important for future screening protocols
2. Personal History of Other Diseases (Z86-Z87)
   - Cardiovascular conditions

- Respiratory disorders
- Digestive system problems
- Previous complications
- Mental health conditions
- Injuries and poisonings

3. History of Medical Treatment (Z92)
   - Past surgical procedures
   - History of medication use
   - Previous radiation therapy
   - Personal history of chemotherapy
   - History of anticoagulation

Coding Guidelines:

Assignment Rules:

- Use only when condition is resolved
- Cannot be used with active conditions
- Must be supported by documentation
- May affect current treatment decisions

Documentation Requirements:

1. Clear statement of previous condition
2. Current status (resolved/inactive)
3. Relevance to present care
4. Any ongoing monitoring needs

Usage in Practice:

- Secondary diagnosis codes
- Risk assessment support
- Treatment planning documentation
- Justification for ongoing surveillance

Common Errors to Avoid:

1. Using history codes for active conditions
2. Failing to link history to current care
3. Missing documentation support
4. Incorrect sequencing with active problems

Impact on Patient Care:

- Guides preventive measures
- Influences treatment choices
- Affects monitoring frequency
- Supports medical necessity

STATUS CODES

Status Codes (Z93-Z99)

Status codes indicate ongoing conditions or situations that affect patient health care. These codes represent current, continuous conditions rather than historical events.

Common Status Categories:

1. Artificial Openings (Z93)
    - Tracheostomy
    - Gastrostomy
    - Colostomy
    - Other artificial openings
2. Device Dependence (Z96-Z97)
    - Cardiac devices
    - Joint replacements
    - Insulin pump
    - Hearing aids
    - Artificial limbs
3. Organ Transplant Status (Z94)
    - Heart transplant
    - Kidney transplant
    - Liver transplant
    - Other organ transplants

FOLLOW-UP CARE

Follow-up care codes describe ongoing care or surveillance after treatment of a condition. They help track continuing care needs and support medical necessity.

Types of Follow-up Care:

Post-Treatment Surveillance

- Cancer follow-up (Z08)
- Other condition monitoring (Z09)
- Regular assessment intervals
- Screening protocols

Aftercare (Z42-Z51)

Specific aftercare needs:

- Wound care
- Device adjustment
- Rehabilitation services
- Medication management
- Therapy services

Documentation Requirements:

For Status Codes:

1. Current condition documentation
2. Ongoing management needs
3. Impact on current care
4. Device/transplant details

For Follow-up Care:

1. Original condition treatment
2. Current care plan
3. Expected duration
4. Monitoring requirements

Coding Guidelines:

Proper Sequencing:

- Status codes typically secondary
- Follow-up codes may be primary
- Must reflect current encounter focus
- Link to related conditions.

Table. Documentation Requirements for Different Z Code Types

Code Type	Required Documentation Elements	Common Errors to Avoid	Supporting Documentation
History Codes	Previous condition, Resolution status, Relevance to current care	Using for active conditions, Missing current relevance	Medical records, Previous treatment notes
Status Codes	Current condition details, Management needs, Device/transplant specifics	Incorrect sequencing, Incomplete documentation	Current exam findings, Device records
Follow-up Codes	Original condition, Treatment provided, Current care plan	Missing treatment history, Incorrect timing documentation	Treatment plans, Progress notes
Screening Codes	Purpose of screening, Test results, Risk factors	Using for symptomatic patients, Missing procedure codes	Orders, Test results

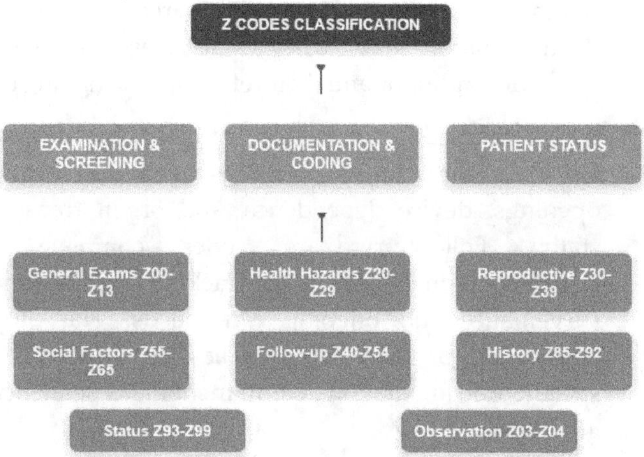

Summary

Z codes represent a fundamental component of medical coding that captures health-related circumstances beyond diseases and injuries. The coding structure encompasses diverse healthcare scenarios, from routine examinations to complex follow-up care protocols. General examinations and screening codes document preventive healthcare measures, while potential health hazard codes address exposure risks and prophylactic interventions. Reproductive health encounters, social circumstances, and personal factors affecting health status are systematically categorized to ensure comprehensive documentation.

The distinction between screening and observation codes is crucial for accurate coding. Screening codes apply to asymptomatic testing scenarios, whereas observation codes document evaluated but ruled-out conditions. Personal history codes serve as vital indicators of past medical conditions that may influence current care decisions, particularly in areas such as previous malignancies, diseases, and medical treatments. These codes require careful attention to documentation that clearly establishes the resolved status of conditions and their relevance to ongoing care.

Status codes differ from history codes by indicating current, continuous conditions such as artificial openings, device dependence, and organ transplant status. Follow-up care codes complete the documentation spectrum by tracking post-treatment surveillance and ongoing care needs. The proper application of these codes relies on adherence to specific documentation requirements and sequencing guidelines.

The systematic organization of Z codes enables healthcare providers to accurately represent the full scope of patient care circumstances, supporting medical necessity and informing treatment decisions. Proper code selection and sequencing are essential for maintaining accurate health records and ensuring appropriate reimbursement.

Multiple Choice Questions

1. Which type of Z codes are used for testing asymptomatic individuals?
   a) Observation codes
   b) Screening codes
   c) Status codes
   d) History codes

2. When a condition is discovered during screening, what happens to the screening code?
   a) It becomes primary
   b) It becomes secondary

c) It is removed
d) It remains unchanged

3. Personal history codes (Z85-Z92) should be used when:
a) Conditions are currently active
b) Conditions are fully resolved
c) Conditions are being treated
d) Conditions are under observation

4. Status codes primarily indicate:
a) Historical conditions
b) Resolved conditions
c) Current, continuous conditions
d) Potential conditions

5. Z codes can be used as:
a) Primary diagnosis only
b) Secondary diagnosis only
c) Both primary and secondary diagnoses
d) Neither primary nor secondary diagnoses

6. Observation codes (Z03-Z04) are used when:
a) A condition is confirmed
b) A condition is being treated
c) A condition is ruled out
d) A condition is screened

7. Which category includes codes for contraceptive management?
a) General Examinations
b) Reproductive Health
c) Follow-up Care
d) Social Circumstances

8. Post-surgical aftercare falls under which Z code category?
   a) Follow-up Care
   b) Status Codes
   c) History Codes
   d) Screening Codes

9. What is required for using observation codes?
   a) Presence of symptoms
   b) Confirmed diagnosis
   c) No symptoms
   d) Clear documentation of ruled-out condition

10. Device dependence status codes include:
    a) Only cardiac devices
    b) Only artificial limbs
    c) Multiple types of devices including cardiac and insulin pumps
    d) Only hearing aids

11. Which code category addresses exposure to communicable diseases?
    a) General Examinations
    b) Potential Health Hazards
    c) Social Circumstances
    d) Follow-up Care

12. Personal history of malignant neoplasms is coded under:
    a) Z93-Z99
    b) Z85
    c) Z03-Z04
    d) Z11-Z13

13. Follow-up care codes Z08-Z09 are primarily used for:
    a) Initial treatment
    b) Post-treatment surveillance
    c) Screening
    d) Device adjustment

14. Which of the following requires status code documentation?
    a) Past conditions
    b) Ruled-out conditions
    c) Current artificial openings
    d) Screening results

15. Social and Personal Circumstances codes (Z55-Z65) include:
    a) Only employment issues
    b) Only educational problems
    c) Only housing concerns
    d) Multiple factors including all of the above

16. Proper documentation for status codes must include:
    a) Historical information only
    b) Current condition and management needs
    c) Future treatment plans only
    d) Past surgical procedures only

17. When using screening codes, the patient should be:
    a) Symptomatic
    b) Asymptomatic
    c) Under treatment
    d) Post-treatment

18. Artificial opening status codes fall under:
    a) Z85-Z92
    b) Z93
    c) Z03-Z04
    d) Z11-Z13

19. For follow-up care coding, documentation must include:
    a) Only original condition
    b) Only current care plan
    c) Both original condition and current care plan
    d) Neither original condition nor care plan

20. Organ transplant status is coded under:
    a) Z93
    b) Z94
    c) Z96
    d) Z99

21. History codes cannot be used with:
    a) Status codes
    b) Follow-up codes
    c) Active conditions
    d) Screening codes

22. Z codes for reproductive health include:
    a) Only pregnancy supervision
    b) Only contraceptive management
    c) Only postpartum care
    d) All of the above

23. Screening codes should be primary when:
    a) A condition is found
    b) Screening is the main reason for visit

c) Multiple conditions exist
d) Treatment is provided

24. Status codes are typically:
    a) Primary diagnosis codes
    b) Secondary diagnosis codes
    c) Not used with other codes
    d) Used only in emergency cases

25. Documentation for history codes must include:
    a) Current active conditions
    b) Future treatment plans
    c) Relevance to present care
    d) Only past procedures

List of Important Questions

1. Explain the fundamental purpose of Z codes in medical coding and their significance in healthcare documentation.
2. How do screening codes differ from observation codes? Discuss with examples.
3. Describe the documentation requirements for using personal history codes and their impact on current patient care.
4. What are the key considerations when coding status codes for artificial openings and device dependence?
5. Discuss the proper sequencing rules for Z codes when used as primary versus secondary diagnoses.
6. Explain the coding guidelines for reproductive health encounters and their various subcategories.
7. How do social and personal circumstance codes contribute to comprehensive patient care documentation?
8. What are the essential elements required in documentation for follow-up care coding?
9. Describe the proper use of Z codes in post-treatment surveillance and aftercare scenarios.
10. How do status codes differ from history codes? Provide examples.
11. Explain the coding guidelines for potential health hazards and preventive measures.
12. What role do Z codes play in documenting organ transplant status and follow-up care?
13. Discuss the importance of proper documentation in supporting the use of Z codes.
14. How are Z codes used in documenting general examinations and screenings?
15. Explain the coding guidelines for documentation of artificial openings and device dependence.

16. What are the key considerations when coding for post-surgical aftercare?
17. How do Z codes support medical necessity documentation?
18. Discuss the proper use of Z codes in documenting family circumstances and social environment problems.
19. What are the common errors to avoid when using history codes?
20. Explain the relationship between Z codes and current active conditions in terms of coding guidelines.

Bibliography

1. Buck CJ. Step-by-Step Medical Coding, 2023 Edition. St. Louis: Elsevier; 2022.
2. Safian SC. Understanding ICD-10-CM and ICD-10-PCS: A Worktext. 5th ed. Burlington: Jones & Bartlett Learning; 2023.
3. World Health Organization. ICD-10: International Statistical Classification of Diseases and Related Health Problems. 10th rev. Geneva: WHO; 2019.
4. Abraham M, Ahlman JT, Boudreau AJ, Connelly JL. CPT 2023 Professional Edition. Chicago: American Medical Association; 2022.
5. Bowman SE. ICD-10-CM and ICD-10-PCS Coding Handbook 2023. Chicago: American Hospital Association Press; 2022.
6. Schmidt M, Schmidt SA, Sandegaard JL, Ehrenstein V, Pedersen L, Sørensen HT. The Danish National Patient Registry: a review of content, data quality, and research potential. Clin Epidemiol. 2015;7:449-90.
7. O'Malley KJ, Cook KF, Price MD, Wildes KR, Hurdle JF, Ashton CM. Measuring diagnoses: ICD code accuracy. Health Serv Res. 2005;40(5):1620-39.
8. Quan H, Li B, Saunders LD, Parsons GA, Nilsson CI, Alibhai A, et al. Assessing validity of ICD-9-CM and ICD-10 administrative data in recording clinical conditions in a unique dually coded database. Health Serv Res. 2008;43(4):1424-41.
9. Centers for Medicare & Medicaid Services. ICD-10-CM Official Guidelines for Coding and Reporting FY 2023. Baltimore: CMS; 2022.
10. Butler RJ, Johnson WG, Baldwin ML. Managing Work Disability: Why First Return to Work Is Not a Measure of Success. ILR Review. 2019;48(3):452-69.

11. Hagland M. The Quality Connection: Documentation Improvement and ICD-10. J AHIMA. 2020;91(6):20-3.
12. Romano PS, Mark DH. Bias in the coding of hospital discharge data and its implications for quality assessment. Med Care. 2020;32(1):81-90.
13. Lucyk K, Tang K, Quan H. Barriers to data quality in the Canadian healthcare system. BMC Health Serv Res. 2017;17(1):766.
14. Hirsch JA, Nicola G, McGinty G, Liu RW, Barr RM, Chittle MD, et al. ICD-10: History and Context. AJNR Am J Neuroradiol. 2016;37(4):596-9.
15. Burns EM, Rigby E, Mamidanna R, Bottle A, Aylin P, Ziprin P, et al. Systematic review of discharge coding accuracy. J Public Health. 2012;34(1):138-48.
16. De Coster C, Quan H, Finlayson A, Gao M, Halfon P, Humphries KH, et al. Identifying priorities in methodological research. BMC Health Serv Res. 2006;6:77.
17. Quan H, Sundararajan V, Halfon P, Fong A, Burnand B, Luthi JC, et al. Coding algorithms for defining comorbidities. Med Care. 2005;43(11):1130-9.
18. Campbell SE, Campbell MK, Grimshaw JM, Walker AE. A systematic review of discharge coding accuracy. J Public Health Med. 2001;23(3):205-11.
19. Nachimson S, Hartley C. The Cost of Implementing ICD-10 Code Sets in Physician Practices. J AHIMA. 2021;92(5):32-6.
20. Centers for Disease Control and Prevention. International Classification of Diseases, Tenth Revision, Clinical Modification (ICD-10-CM). Atlanta: CDC; 2023.

CHAPTER 10

DOCUMENTATION REQUIREMENTS

Author

Mr. Gourab Saha, Assistant Professor, Department of Pharmaceutics, College of Pharmaceutical Sciences, Berhampur, Mohada, Odisha, India

Abstract

Medical record documentation forms the foundation of medical coding and billing, encompassing essential components that ensure accurate coding, proper reimbursement, and quality patient care. The documentation process starts with patient demographics and progresses through detailed clinical documentation including chief complaint, history of present illness, past medical history, family history, social history, and review of systems. Physical examination findings and assessment/plan complete the basic clinical documentation. Supporting documentation includes laboratory results, diagnostic imaging reports, consultation notes, operative reports, pathology findings, nursing notes, progress notes, and various medical orders. The query process facilitates communication between providers and coders to clarify documentation ambiguities through concurrent or retrospective queries. Clinical Documentation Improvement (CDI) programs systematically enhance documentation quality through concurrent review, provider education, quality monitoring, and compliance oversight. Regulatory compliance requirements govern documentation practices, including HIPAA regulations, Medicare/Medicaid requirements, medical necessity documentation, coding compliance, and electronic health record standards. Healthcare organizations must maintain robust audit programs and provide ongoing education to ensure documentation meets all applicable standards while protecting patient privacy and security.

Keywords: *Medical Documentation; Clinical Coding; Documentation Compliance; Clinical Queries; Documentation Improvement*

Learning Objectives

After completion of the chapter, the student should be able to:

- Identify and describe the essential components of medical record documentation, including basic elements and supporting documentation requirements.
- Demonstrate understanding of the query process and its role in clarifying documentation ambiguities through both concurrent and retrospective approaches.
- Analyze the key components and strategies of Clinical Documentation Improvement programs and their impact on documentation quality.
- Apply compliance requirements in medical documentation, including regulatory standards, medical necessity documentation, and coding compliance.
- Evaluate documentation integrity in electronic health records, including proper use of templates, authentication requirements, and copy-paste policies.
- Understand privacy and security compliance measures in medical documentation, including access controls and breach response protocols.

MEDICAL RECORD COMPONENTS

Medical record documentation is the foundation of medical coding and billing. A well-documented medical record serves as the primary tool for justifying medical necessity and supporting the codes selected for billing purposes. Let's explore each component in detail.

Basic components

Patient Demographics:

The cornerstone of any medical record begins with accurate patient demographics. This section must include the patient's full legal name, date of birth, gender, address, contact information, insurance details, and emergency contact information. For billing purposes, accurate demographic information is crucial as errors in this section can lead to claim denials and delayed reimbursement.

Chief Complaint (CC):

The chief complaint represents the patient's primary reason for seeking medical attention, expressed preferably in the patient's own words. This component drives the entire encounter and must be clearly documented. For example, instead of simply noting "stomach pain," a proper chief complaint would read "Patient states: 'I've had severe upper abdominal pain for the past three days.'" The chief complaint helps establish medical necessity for the visit and subsequent procedures or tests.

History of Present Illness (HPI):

The HPI is a chronological description of the development of the patient's present illness from the first sign or symptom to the present. This section must include the following elements:

Location: Where is the sign or symptom?

Quality: What is the characteristic of the sign or symptom?

Severity: How severe is the sign or symptom?

Duration: How long has the sign or symptom been present?

Timing: When does the sign or symptom occur? Context: What circumstances are associated with the sign or symptom?
Modifying factors: What makes the sign or symptom better or worse?
Associated signs and symptoms: What other symptoms are present?

Table. Documentation Components and Required Elements

Component	Required Elements	Documentation Impact
Patient Demographics	- Full legal name - Date of birth - Gender - Address - Insurance details - Emergency contacts	Essential for billing and identification
Chief Complaint	- Primary reason for visit - Patient's own words - Onset timing	Establishes medical necessity
History of Present Illness	- Location- Quality - Severity- Duration - Timing - Context - Modifying factors - Associated symptoms	Determines E/M level and supports medical decision-making
Physical Examination	- Vital signs - System -specific findings - Positive/negative results	Supports diagnosis and treatment plans

Past Medical History (PMH):

PMH encompasses all significant medical events in the patient's life, including previous illnesses, injuries, surgeries, hospitalizations, and current medications. This section should also document allergies and adverse reactions to medications. For coding purposes, past medical history can significantly impact the selection of diagnosis codes and help establish medical necessity for certain procedures.

Family History:

This component documents significant health conditions present in the patient's blood relatives. It's particularly important for identifying genetic predispositions and risk factors. Coders should pay attention to family history as it may support the medical necessity of preventive services or diagnostic testing.

Social History:

Social history includes relevant aspects of the patient's life that may impact their health, such as:

- Occupation and workplace exposures
- Living conditions and arrangements
- Marriage status
- Substance use (tobacco, alcohol, recreational drugs)
- Diet and exercise habits
- Travel history when relevant

Review of Systems (ROS):

The ROS is a systematic review of body systems obtained through a series of questions seeking to identify signs and symptoms that the patient may be experiencing. The systems typically covered include:

- Constitutional symptoms
- Eyes
- Ears, Nose, Mouth, and Throat

- Cardiovascular
- Respiratory
- Gastrointestinal
- Genitourinary
- Musculoskeletal
- Integumentary
- Neurological
- Psychiatric
- Endocrine
- Hematologic/Lymphatic
- Allergic/Immunologic

Physical Examination:

This section documents the provider's objective findings through observation, palpation, percussion, and auscultation. The extent of the examination can range from problem-focused to comprehensive, depending on the nature of the visit. Documentation should be specific and include both positive and relevant negative findings.

Assessment and Plan:

The assessment provides the provider's conclusions about the patient's condition, including diagnoses and differential diagnoses. The plan outlines the proposed treatment, including medications, procedures, additional testing, referrals, and follow-up care. This section is crucial for code selection as it often contains the definitive diagnoses used for coding.

Essential documentation elements

Date of Service:

Every entry in the medical record must be dated. This includes the date and, when relevant, the time of service. This is particularly important for procedures and time-based services.

Provider Identification and Signatures:

All entries must be authenticated by the provider through a legible signature with credentials. Electronic signatures must comply with CMS and organizational policies. Each provider involved in the patient's care should be clearly identifiable.

Patient Identification:

Every page of the medical record should include patient identification to prevent documentation errors and comply with legal requirements. This typically includes the patient's name and a unique identifier like a medical record number.

Legibility:

Whether handwritten or electronic, all documentation must be legible to any reader. Illegible documentation can lead to medical errors and denied claims. Electronic Health Records (EHRs) have largely addressed this issue, but it remains important for any handwritten notes or amendments.

Clear Documentation of Procedures:

When procedures are performed, documentation must include:

Specific name of the procedure

Anatomical site and laterality

Any complications or unusual circumstances

Medical necessity justification

Informed consent when required

Time Documentation:

Time documentation is essential for certain services, particularly:

Evaluation and Management services when counseling dominates the visit

Critical care services

Prolonged services
Time-based procedures

Authentication of Entries:

All entries must be properly authenticated following organizational policies and regulatory requirements. This includes:
Original signatures or electronic authentication
Date and time of authentication
Proper handling of late entries or amendments
Documentation of verbal orders

SUPPORTING DOCUMENTATION

Supporting documentation in medical records serves as crucial evidence that validates the medical necessity, appropriateness, and quality of healthcare services provided. This documentation forms the backbone of accurate medical coding and successful claim submissions.

Types of Supporting Documentation

Laboratory Results:

Laboratory results provide objective clinical data that supports diagnosis codes and medical necessity. Documentation must include:

- Order date and provider information
- Test name and methodology
- Reference ranges and actual results
- Collection date and time
- Any critical values and provider notification
- Interpretation and clinical significance when required

For coding purposes, laboratory results often support the specificity of diagnosis codes and the medical necessity of follow-up services or procedures.

Diagnostic Imaging Reports:

Imaging documentation requires:

- Study type and anatomical area
- Technique and contrast use
- Detailed findings and impressions
- Comparison with prior studies when available
- Technical quality and limitations
- Recommendations for follow-up

These reports are essential for supporting procedural codes and demonstrating medical necessity for subsequent treatments or procedures.

Consultation Reports:

Consultation documentation must include:

- Reason for consultation
- Specialist's detailed findings
- Diagnostic impressions
- Treatment recommendations
- Communication with referring provider

Proper consultation documentation supports both the medical necessity of the consultation and any subsequent specialty care.

Operative Reports:

Operative reports require comprehensive documentation including:

Preoperative Diagnosis:

he condition that indicated the need for surgery, supporting medical necessity.

Postoperative Diagnosis:

Findings during surgery that confirm or modify the preoperative diagnosis.

Procedure Description:

- Detailed step-by-step account of the procedure
- Surgical approach and technique
- Anatomical structures involved

- Any complications or unusual circumstances
- Surgical findings
- Estimated blood loss
- Specimens removed
- Implants or devices used

This detailed documentation is crucial for accurate CPT code selection and modifier usage.

Pathology Reports:

Pathology documentation must include:

- Specimen description and source
- Gross examination findings
- Microscopic examination results
- Diagnosis or conclusion
- Any additional testing performed
- Correlation with clinical findings

These reports often provide the highest level of diagnostic specificity required for accurate ICD-10-CM coding.

Nursing Notes:

Nursing documentation provides valuable supporting information:

- Patient assessment findings
- Medication administration
- Treatment responses
- Patient education
- Care coordination
- Changes in patient status

While not directly used for coding, nursing notes often provide context and support for services billed.

Progress Notes:

Progress notes should document:

Clinical Progress:

- Response to treatments
- Changes in symptoms or condition

- New problems or complications
- Status of chronic conditions

Treatment Modifications:

- Changes in medication or treatment plans
- Rationale for changes
- Patient response to modifications

Follow-up Plans:

- Next appointment scheduling
- Referrals made
- Testing ordered
- Modified treatment goals

Orders and Prescriptions: Documentation must include:

- Complete medication orders including dose, route, and frequency
- Diagnostic test orders with clinical indicators
- Treatment orders with specific parameters
- Referral orders with reason for referral
- Patient instructions and education

Documentation Guidelines for Supporting Documents

Medical Necessity Support: All supporting documentation should clearly establish medical necessity through:

- Clear connection between symptoms and diagnostic tests
- Rational progression of treatment decisions
- Evidence-based care protocols
- Documentation of failed conservative treatment when required

Specific Requirements for Procedures: Procedure documentation must include:

- Indication for the procedure
- Informed consent
- Time and duration when relevant
- Specific techniques and approaches used

- Complications and their management
- Post-procedure care instructions

Documentation for E/M Services: Supporting documentation for E/M services requires:

- Clear demonstration of service level components
- Time documentation when applicable
- Medical decision-making elements
- Coordination of care activities

Requirements for Diagnostic Testing: Documentation must support:

- Medical necessity for ordered tests
- Specific signs or symptoms indicating testing
- Prior test results when relevant
- How results will impact patient care

QUERY PROCESS

The query process represents a vital communication bridge between healthcare providers and coding professionals. This systematic approach ensures accurate code assignment and maintains documentation integrity. Understanding and implementing an effective query process is essential for successful medical coding practice.

Purpose of Clinical Queries

Documentation clarification stands as the cornerstone of the query process. When medical records contain ambiguous, conflicting, or incomplete information, coding professionals must seek clarification to ensure accurate code assignment. For instance, a provider might document "pneumonia" without specifying the type or causative organism. In such cases, a query becomes necessary to obtain the specific information required for the most accurate ICD-10-CM code assignment.

Clinical queries also serve to validate documented

diagnoses when clinical indicators appear inconsistent with the stated conditions. Consider a scenario where a provider documents acute respiratory failure, but the clinical indicators such as blood gases, respiratory rate, and oxygen saturation appear normal. This disconnect would necessitate a query to ensure proper documentation supports the diagnosis.

Table. Query Types and Characteristics

Query Type	Timing	Advantages	Challenges	Best Used For
Concurrent	During patient stay	- Immediate access to provider - Fresh clinical details- Quick resolution	- Provider availability - Time constraints	- Critical clarifications - Complex cases
Retrospective	After discharge	- Complete record review - Thorough analysis	- Delayed responses- Memory limitations	- Audit preparation- Quality reviews
Verbal	Any time	- Quick resolution - Direct communication	- Documentation needs - No permanent record	- Simple clarifications - Urgent situations
Written	Any time	- Clear audit trail - Detailed explanation	- Response delays- Format constraints	- Complex queries - Compliance issues

Types of Queries

Healthcare facilities employ several types of queries, each serving specific purposes and situations. Understanding when and how to use each type maximizes the effectiveness of the query process.

Concurrent queries occur while the patient is still receiving care or shortly after discharge. These real-time queries offer significant advantages, including immediate access to the treating provider and fresh clinical details. For example, during an inpatient stay, a coding professional might notice missing specificity in a diabetes diagnosis and can quickly obtain clarification while the provider is still actively managing the patient's care.

Retrospective queries, conducted after the patient's discharge, often arise during coding review or audit preparation. While these queries present challenges such as delayed responses and potential memory limitations, they remain crucial for maintaining documentation accuracy. A coding professional might initiate a retrospective query when reviewing records for a quarterly audit and discovering insufficient documentation for a reported procedure.

Verbal queries involve direct communication with providers and prove especially useful in urgent situations or for simple clarifications. However, proper documentation of these verbal exchanges remains crucial. When using verbal queries, coding professionals should always follow up with written documentation to maintain a clear audit trail.

Written queries represent the most formal and trackable communication method. These queries require careful construction to ensure clarity while avoiding leading questions. A well-constructed written query includes relevant clinical indicators, presents multiple reasonable options, and allows providers to exercise their clinical judgment.

Query Best Practices

Successful query processes rely on adherence to established best practices. Non-leading questions form the foundation of compliant queries. Rather than suggesting specific diagnoses, queries should present multiple reasonable options based on clinical indicators. For example, instead of asking, "Was this viral pneumonia?" a proper query might ask, "Please specify the type of pneumonia based on the following clinical indicators..."

Clinical indicators play a crucial role in query construction. Every query should reference specific findings, test results, or treatment protocols that prompted the need for clarification. This approach helps providers understand the context and importance of the query while supporting their clinical decision-making process.

Query timing requires careful consideration of various factors, including billing deadlines, provider availability, and clinical relevance. While concurrent queries often prove most effective, circumstances sometimes necessitate retrospective queries. The key lies in maintaining a balance between timely coding and accurate documentation.

Query Process Management

Effective query management requires a structured approach with clear policies and procedures. Healthcare organizations should establish standard timeframes for query responses and create escalation protocols for unaddressed queries. Regular monitoring of query metrics helps identify trends and opportunities for documentation improvement.

Education plays a vital role in query process success. Both coding professionals and healthcare providers need ongoing training in proper query construction, documentation requirements, and compliance standards. This educational component helps reduce the need for queries over time by promoting better initial documentation.

Query Resolution and Follow-up

The query process doesn't end with obtaining provider responses. Proper documentation of query resolution includes updating medical records, modifying codes as needed, and maintaining a clear audit trail. Quality review of resolved queries helps identify patterns and opportunities for documentation improvement.

Regular analysis of query patterns can reveal common documentation deficiencies and guide targeted provider education efforts. For instance, if multiple queries consistently address the same documentation issue, this might indicate a need for focused education on that specific topic.

CLINICAL DOCUMENTATION IMPROVEMENT

Clinical Documentation Improvement represents a systematic approach to enhancing the quality, precision, and completeness of medical record documentation. This comprehensive process supports accurate code assignment, appropriate reimbursement, and quality patient care metrics.

Understanding CDI Program Components

A successful CDI program requires careful structuring and implementation. At its core, the program must align clinical documentation with coding requirements while maintaining the integrity of the medical record. This begins with establishing a dedicated CDI team, typically comprising registered nurses, coding professionals, and clinical documentation specialists who work collaboratively with healthcare providers.

The foundation of any CDI program rests on four key pillars:

The first pillar involves concurrent record review, where CDI specialists examine documentation during patient encounters. This real-time review allows for immediate identification and resolution of documentation gaps, reducing the need for retrospective queries and preventing delays in the revenue cycle.

The second pillar focuses on provider education. This involves regular training sessions, one-on-one consultations, and feedback mechanisms that help physicians understand documentation requirements without compromising their clinical workflow.

The third pillar encompasses quality monitoring through regular audits and performance metrics. This continuous assessment helps identify areas for improvement and measures the program's effectiveness.

The fourth pillar consists of compliance oversight, ensuring all documentation practices align with regulatory requirements and industry standards.

CDI Strategies for Success

Effective CDI programs employ various strategies to achieve optimal documentation outcomes. The concurrent review process stands as perhaps the most crucial strategy. During these reviews, CDI specialists evaluate documentation for:

Clinical Validity:

Ensuring documented diagnoses are supported by

clinical indicators, laboratory results, and treatment plans. For instance, when a provider documents sepsis, the documentation should reflect systemic inflammatory response syndrome (SIRS) criteria and appropriate treatment protocols.

Diagnostic Specificity:

Promoting the highest level of diagnostic precision possible. Rather than documenting "pneumonia," the record should specify the type, causative organism if known, and any associated complications.

Treatment Justification:

Supporting medical necessity for all procedures and services through clear documentation of clinical indicators and failed conservative treatments when applicable.

Provider engagement represents another critical strategy. Successful CDI programs develop strong relationships with medical staff through:

Regular Communication:

Establishing consistent channels for feedback and discussion about documentation needs. This might include monthly meetings, newsletters, or electronic communication platforms.

Educational Resources:

Creating easily accessible reference materials, including documentation tips, common terminology requirements, and clinical indicators for frequently encountered conditions.

Performance Feedback:

Providing individual and group feedback on documentation patterns, including areas of excellence and opportunities for improvement.

Common Documentation Challenges

Understanding common documentation challenges helps CDI programs focus their improvement efforts effectively. Several recurring issues often surface in medical records:

Diagnosis Specificity:

Many providers document conditions without the level of detail required for accurate coding. For example, documenting "chronic kidney disease" without specifying the stage limits code assignment and potentially affects quality metrics.

Clinical Linkages:

Providers sometimes fail to establish clear relationships between conditions, complications, and underlying causes. The connection between diabetes and its manifestations, for instance, must be explicitly documented.

Temporal Factors:

Documentation sometimes lacks clear timing elements, making it difficult to determine when conditions developed or resolved. This becomes particularly important in distinguishing present-on-admission conditions from hospital-acquired complications.

Measuring CDI Success

Effective CDI programs require robust measurement systems to evaluate their impact. Key performance indicators typically include:

Case Mix Index (CMI) Changes: Tracking changes in CMI helps measure the program's effectiveness in capturing appropriate complexity levels.

Query Response Rates: Monitoring provider responses to queries indicates engagement levels and identifies areas needing additional focus.

Documentation Quality Scores: Regular audits of medical records provide quantitative measures of documentation improvement over time.

Financial Impact: Analyzing changes in reimbursement patterns and denial rates helps justify program investment and identify areas for expansion

Table. CDI Program Performance Metrics

Metric Category	Specific Measures	Target Goals	Monitoring Frequency
Documentation Quality	- Accuracy rate - Completeness score - Query rate	- >95% accuracy - >90% completeness - <15% query rate	Monthly
Financial Impact	- Case Mix Index - Reimbursement changes - Denial rates	- CMI improvement - Reduced denials - Increased revenue	Quarterly
Provider Engagement	- Query response rate Documentation timeliness - Education attendance	- >90% response rate - <24hr documentation - >80% attendance	Monthly
Compliance	-Authentication compliance - Template usage - Amendment rates	- 100% authentication - Appropriate usage <5% amendment rate	Weekly

COMPLIANCE REQUIREMENTS

Healthcare documentation compliance encompasses a complex framework of regulatory requirements, professional standards, and legal obligations. Understanding and adhering to these compliance requirements is fundamental for healthcare organizations, providers, and coding professionals to maintain integrity in healthcare delivery and billing practices.

Regulatory Framework

The healthcare industry operates under multiple regulatory bodies and legislative acts that govern documentation practices. The Health Insurance Portability and Accountability Act (HIPAA) serves as a cornerstone of healthcare documentation compliance, establishing standards for protected health information (PHI) privacy and security. Organizations must maintain strict protocols for accessing, storing, and transmitting medical records while ensuring patient confidentiality.

Medicare and Medicaid requirements add another layer of complexity to documentation compliance. The Centers for Medicare & Medicaid Services (CMS) establishes specific documentation guidelines that providers must follow to support medical necessity and claim submission. These guidelines affect everything from evaluation and management service documentation to proper procedure documentation requirements.

Documentation Integrity

Medical record integrity forms the foundation of compliance requirements. Each entry in the medical record must be complete, accurate, and timely. Providers must authenticate their documentation through signatures, whether physical or electronic, and include their credentials and the date of service. Any amendments or corrections to the medical record must follow strict protocols, including maintaining the original entry while clearly identifying the correction, the person making it, and the date of modification.

Time-based documentation requires particular attention to compliance. When services are billed based on time, such as critical care or prolonged services, documentation must clearly reflect the time spent, specific activities performed, and the medical necessity for the duration of service. This documentation should be contemporaneous and specific enough to support the time-based billing codes selected.

Medical Necessity Documentation

Medical necessity represents a crucial compliance requirement that affects both documentation and reimbursement. Documentation must clearly establish the need for each service, procedure, or test ordered. This includes:

Clinical Rationale:

Documentation should clearly articulate the clinical reasoning behind diagnostic tests, treatments, and procedures. For example, when ordering advanced imaging studies, providers should document specific signs, symptoms, or conditions that necessitate the study.

Failed Conservative Treatment:

When applicable, documentation should reflect previous treatment attempts and their outcomes. This becomes particularly important for surgical procedures or advanced therapeutic interventions.

Risk Assessment:

Documentation should include the provider's assessment of potential risks and benefits, especially for invasive procedures or high-risk treatments.

Coding Compliance

Documentation must support the codes selected for billing purposes. This includes both diagnosis and procedure codes. The documented diagnostic statement must be clearly supported by clinical findings, test results, and the assessment and plan. Similarly, procedure documentation must include all required elements to support the CPT or HCPCS code selected.

Professional Services:

Documentation for professional services must clearly delineate:

- The specific service provided
- The provider's direct participation
- The time spent when relevant
- The medical decision-making process
- Any coordination of care activities

Facility Services:

Facility documentation requirements include:

- Resources utilized
- Level of care provided
- Support staff involvement
- Equipment and supplies used
- Duration of services

Teaching Physician Requirements

Teaching facilities face additional documentation requirements. When residents or fellows participate in patient care, documentation must clearly identify:

The teaching physician's presence and participation in key portions of the service

Specific involvement in medical decision-making Personal review of the patient and findings

Agreement or disagreement with resident documentation
Independent verification of critical elements

Electronic Health Record Compliance

As healthcare organizations increasingly rely on electronic health records (EHR), specific compliance requirements apply to electronic documentation:

Authentication Requirements: Electronic signatures must meet CMS and organizational standards for authenticity and security.

Copy-and-Paste Policies:

Organizations must establish and enforce policies regarding the appropriate use of copied information within the EHR, ensuring that each entry reflects current, accurate information.

Template Usage:

While templates can promote documentation efficiency, they must be used appropriately to reflect individual patient encounters rather than generic information.

Audit Requirements

Healthcare organizations must maintain robust audit programs to ensure documentation compliance. These programs should include:

Regular Internal Audits:

Systematic review of documentation practices to identify potential compliance issues before they become problematic.

External Audit Preparation:

Maintenance of documentation that can withstand scrutiny from external auditors, including Medicare Administrative Contractors (MACs) and Recovery Audit

Contractors (RACs).

Corrective Action Planning: Development and implementation of improvement plans based on audit findings.

Education and Training

Maintaining documentation compliance requires ongoing education and training efforts:

Initial Training:

New providers and staff members must receive comprehensive training on documentation requirements specific to their roles.

Continuing Education:

Regular updates on changing requirements and identified areas for improvement help maintain compliance standards.

Focused Training:

Additional education targeting specific documentation deficiencies identified through audits or quality reviews.

Privacy and Security Compliance

Documentation compliance extends to protecting patient information:

Access Controls: Implementation of appropriate restrictions on who can access medical records and under what circumstances.

Security Measures: Maintenance of physical and electronic safeguards to protect patient information from unauthorized access or disclosure.

Breach Response: Development and maintenance of protocols for responding to potential privacy or security breaches.

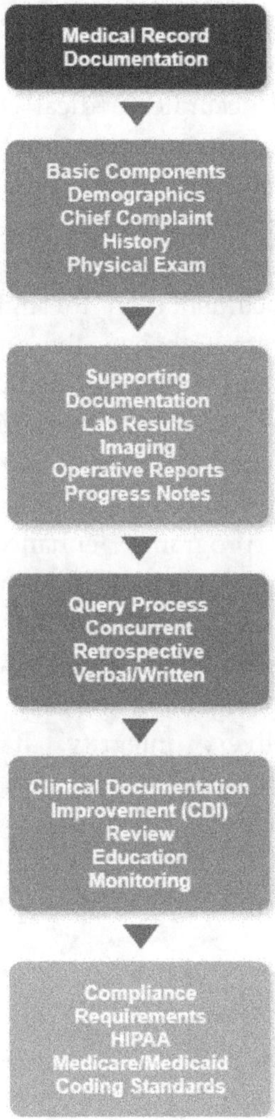
Medical Record
Documentation
Basic Components
Demographics
Chief Complaint
History
Physical Exam
Supporting
Documentation
Lab Results
Imaging
Operative Reports
Progress Notes
Query Process
Concurrent
Retrospective
Verbal/Written
Clinical Documentation
Improvement (CDI)
Review
Education
Monitoring
Compliance
Requirements
HIPAA
Medicare/Medicaid
Coding Standards

Summary

Medical record documentation serves as the cornerstone of accurate medical coding and billing, requiring meticulous attention to detail and compliance with established standards. The basic components, from patient demographics to assessment and plan, provide the framework for documenting patient care. Supporting documentation through various reports and notes strengthens the medical record's completeness and validates medical necessity. The query process enables effective communication between providers and coders to resolve documentation uncertainties. Clinical Documentation Improvement programs enhance documentation quality through systematic review, education, and monitoring processes. Compliance requirements ensure documentation meets regulatory standards while protecting patient privacy and maintaining healthcare delivery integrity. It is essential for healthcare providers, coders, and organizations to maintain accurate records, support proper reimbursement, and deliver quality patient care by understanding and implementing these documentation principles.

Multiple Choice Questions

1. Which component of medical record documentation serves as the primary reason for the patient's visit?
   a) Past Medical History
   b) Chief Complaint
   c) Review of Systems
   d) Physical Examination

2. An effective HPI (History of Present Illness) must include:
   a) Only location and duration
   b) At least 8 elements
   c) Only severity and timing
   d) Family medical history

3. The ROS (Review of Systems) typically includes documentation of:
   a) Only major body systems
   b) 14 body systems
   c) 5 body systems
   d) Only affected systems

4. Which type of query is conducted while the patient is still receiving care?
   a) Retrospective query
   b) Concurrent query
   c) Written query
   d) Post-discharge query

5. In CDI programs, what does CMI stand for?
   a) Clinical Management Index
   b) Case Mix Index

c) Clinical Measure Index
d) Care Management Initiative

6. Laboratory result documentation must include:
a) Only test results
b) Only reference ranges
c) Provider information and test methodology
d) All of the above

7. Which documentation element is crucial for time-based billing codes?
a) Provider signature only
b) Date of service only
c) Specific time documentation
d) Patient demographics

8. What is required for proper authentication of medical record entries?
a) Date only
b) Provider signature only
c) Time only
d) Provider signature, credentials, and date

9. The query process should avoid:
a) Written documentation
b) Leading questions
c) Clinical indicators
d) Multiple options

10. What is a key purpose of supporting documentation?
a) Validate medical necessity
b) Replace primary documentation

c) Eliminate need for queries
d) Reduce documentation requirements

11. A successful CDI program primarily focuses on:
    a) Billing only
    b) Coding only
    c) Documentation improvement
    d) Patient scheduling

12. Which is NOT a type of query?
    a) Concurrent
    b) Retrospective
    c) Predictive
    d) Verbal

13. Social history documentation should include:
    a) Only occupation
    b) Only substance use
    c) Multiple aspects of patient's life
    d) Only marital status

14. Medical necessity documentation must demonstrate:
    a) Only diagnosis
    b) Only treatment plan
    c) Clinical rationale for services
    d) Only insurance information

15. Electronic health record compliance requires:
    a) Only electronic signatures
    b) No templates
    c) Specific authentication standards
    d) Paper backup only

16. Progress notes should document:
    a) Only new problems
    b) Only medications
    c) Clinical progress and treatment modifications
    d) Only lab results

17. Operative reports must include:
    a) Only postoperative diagnosis
    b) Only surgical technique
    c) Comprehensive procedure description
    d) Only estimated blood loss

18. The foundation of medical coding and billing is:
    a) Insurance verification
    b) Medical record documentation
    c) Patient scheduling
    d) Provider credentials

19. Which is NOT a pillar of CDI programs?
    a) Concurrent record review
    b) Provider education
    c) Patient satisfaction
    d) Quality monitoring

20. HIPAA primarily governs:
    a) Billing procedures
    b) Protected health information
    c) Staffing requirements
    d) Treatment protocols

21. Teaching physician documentation must show:
    a) Only resident involvement
    b) Only independent verification

c) Presence and participation in key portions
d) Only student observation

22. Pathology reports must include:
a) Only microscopic findings
b) Only gross examination
c) Both gross and microscopic findings
d) Only specimen source

23. What is required for amendments to medical records?
a) Only new date
b) Only new signature
c) Original entry preservation and clear identification of changes
d) Complete deletion of original entry

24. Clinical indicators in queries should:
a) Suggest specific diagnoses
b) Support the need for clarification
c) Be omitted
d) Only include lab values

25. Documentation compliance audits should be:
a) Done once yearly
b) Never done
c) Regular and systematic
d) Done only when required by external agencies

List of Important Questions

1. Explain the significance of medical record documentation in medical coding and billing.
2. Describe the eight essential elements of History of Present Illness (HPI) and their importance.
3. How does the Review of Systems (ROS) contribute to comprehensive medical documentation?
4. Compare and contrast concurrent and retrospective queries in medical documentation.
5. Discuss the role of Clinical Documentation Improvement (CDI) programs in healthcare organizations.
6. What are the key components of supporting documentation, and how do they validate medical necessity?
7. Analyze the importance of query construction and best practices in the documentation process.
8. Explain the compliance requirements for electronic health record documentation.
9. What are the essential elements of operative report documentation?
10. Discuss the role of clinical indicators in medical necessity documentation.
11. How do teaching physician requirements differ from standard documentation requirements?
12. Explain the significance of authentication in medical record documentation.
13. What are the key considerations for maintaining documentation integrity in electronic health records?
14. Describe the components and importance of pathology report documentation.
15. How does HIPAA compliance affect medical record documentation practices?
16. Discuss the role of audit programs in maintaining documentation compliance.

17. What are the essential elements of progress note documentation?
18. Explain the importance of time documentation in medical records.
19. How do CDI specialists contribute to improving documentation quality?
20. Discuss the significance of medical necessity documentation in the healthcare revenue cycle.

Bibliography

1. O'Malley KJ, Cook KF, Price MD, Wildes KR, Hurdle JF, Ashton CM. Measuring diagnoses: ICD code accuracy. Health Serv Res. 2005;40(5):1620-39.
2. Hripcsak G, Vawdrey DK, Fred MR, Bostwick SB. Use of electronic clinical documentation: time spent and team interactions. J Am Med Inform Assoc. 2011;18(2):112-7.
3. Edwards ST, Neri PM, Volk LA, Schiff GD, Bates DW. Association of note quality and quality of care: a cross-sectional study. BMJ Qual Saf. 2014;23(5):406-13.
4. Towers AL. Clinical documentation improvement: a physician perspective. Clin Colon Rectal Surg. 2013;26(3):124-7.
5. Rosenbloom ST, Denny JC, Xu H, Lorenzi N, Stead WW, Johnson KB. Data from clinical notes: a perspective on the tension between structure and flexible documentation. J Am Med Inform Assoc. 2011;18(2):181-6.
6. Kripalani S, LeFevre F, Phillips CO, Williams MV, Basaviah P, Baker DW. Deficits in communication and information transfer between hospital-based and primary care physicians. JAMA. 2007;297(8):831-41.
7. Singh H, Giardina TD, Meyer AN, Forjuoh SN, Reis MD, Thomas EJ. Types and origins of diagnostic errors in primary care settings. JAMA Intern Med. 2013;173(6):418-25.
8. Siegler EL, Adelman R. Copy and paste: a remediable hazard of electronic health records. Am J Med. 2009;122(6):495-6.
9. Weiskopf NG, Weng C. Methods and dimensions of electronic health record data quality assessment: enabling reuse for clinical research. J Am Med Inform Assoc. 2013;20(1):144-51.

10. Adler-Milstein J, Jha AK. HITECH Act drove large gains in hospital electronic health record adoption. Health Aff (Millwood). 2017;36(8):1416-22.
11. Bowman S. Impact of electronic health record systems on information integrity: quality and safety implications. Perspect Health Inf Manag. 2013;10(Fall):1c.
12. Stead WW, Lin HS, editors. Computational technology for effective health care: immediate steps and strategic directions. Washington (DC): National Academies Press; 2009.
13. Dean BB, Lam J, Natoli JL, Butler Q, Aguilar D, Nordyke RJ. Review: use of electronic medical records for health outcomes research. Med Care Res Rev. 2009;66(6):611-38.
14. Hayrinen K, Saranto K, Nykanen P. Definition, structure, content, use and impacts of electronic health records: a review of the research literature. Int J Med Inform. 2008;77(5):291-304.
15. Kushniruk AW, Bates DW, Bainbridge M, Househ MS, Borycki EM. National efforts to improve health information system safety in Canada, the United States of America and England. Int J Med Inform. 2013;82(5):e149-60.
16. Holroyd-Leduc JM, Lorenzetti D, Straus SE, Sykes L, Quan H. The impact of the electronic medical record on structure, process, and outcomes within primary care: a systematic review of the evidence. J Am Med Inform Assoc. 2011;18(6):732-7.
17. Chan KS, Fowles JB, Weiner JP. Electronic health records and the reliability and validity of quality measures: a review of the literature. Med Care Res Rev. 2010;67(5):503-27.
18. Sittig DF, Singh H. A new sociotechnical model for studying health information technology in complex

adaptive healthcare systems. Qual Saf Health Care. 2010;19(Suppl 3):i68-74.

19. Romano MJ, Stafford RS. Electronic health records and clinical decision support systems: impact on national ambulatory care quality. Arch Intern Med. 2011;171(10):897-903.
20. Ash JS, Berg M, Coiera E. Some unintended consequences of information technology in health care: the nature of patient care information system-related errors. J Am Med Inform Assoc. 2004;11(2):104-12.

CHAPTER 11

CODING ETHICS AND COMPLIANCE

Author

Mrs. Jeslin D, Associate Professor, Department of Pharmaceutics, Faculty of Pharmacy, Sree Balaji Medical College and Hospital Campus, Bharath Institute of Higher Education & Research, Chennai, Tamil Nadu, India

Abstract

Medical coding ethics, compliance, and documentation requirements form the foundation of healthcare revenue integrity and regulatory adherence. Ethical coding practices demand truthfulness, accuracy, and professional integrity in code assignment based solely on clinical documentation. The comprehensive framework encompasses HIPAA compliance for protecting patient health information through administrative, physical, and technical safeguards. Documentation requirements establish standards for clear, consistent, and authenticated medical records that support code assignment and medical necessity. Fraud prevention strategies include systematic controls, monitoring systems, and compliance programs to identify and prevent fraudulent coding practices like upcoding and unbundling. Quality assurance programs implement regular monitoring, performance metrics, and error analysis to maintain coding accuracy and compliance. The framework addresses security incidents, breach notifications, and business associate relationships while emphasizing ongoing education, documentation retention, and compliance monitoring. Proper query processes ensure clarification of unclear documentation through objective communication. A structured approach to quality assurance incorporates performance metrics, error analysis, educational support, and continuous program improvement to maintain high coding standards. The integration of technology, team collaboration, and success measurements ensures sustained quality in medical coding operations while adhering to external regulatory requirements and professional standards.

Keywords: *Medical coding ethics; HIPAA compliance; Documentation standards; Fraud prevention; Quality assurance*

Learning Objectives

After completion of the chapter, the student should be able to:

- Demonstrate understanding of fundamental coding ethics principles and their application in daily coding practices
- Explain HIPAA compliance requirements and implement appropriate safeguards for protected health information
- Identify common types of coding fraud and develop effective prevention strategies
- Apply proper documentation standards and query protocols in medical record management
- Design and implement comprehensive quality assurance programs for coding accuracy
- Evaluate coding practices for compliance with federal regulations and professional standards

CODING ETHICS GUIDELINES

Ethics in medical coding forms the cornerstone of healthcare revenue integrity and compliance. Coding professionals must adhere to strict ethical principles that govern their daily practice, ensuring accuracy, honesty, and accountability in all coding decisions.

Fundamental Principles of Coding Ethics

The foundation of coding ethics rests on several core principles that guide professional practice. Truthfulness serves as the primary principle, requiring coding professionals to report only documented clinical facts without manipulation or assumption. This commitment to truth extends beyond mere technical accuracy to encompass the spirit and intent of coding guidelines.

Integrity in coding practice demands that professionals assign codes based solely on clinical documentation, regardless of potential financial implications. This means resisting any pressure to "optimize" coding for financial gain when such optimization would compromise accuracy. For instance, when documentation supports multiple interpretation possibilities, coding professionals must choose the most clinically appropriate option rather than the most financially advantageous one.

Professional integrity also includes maintaining current knowledge of coding guidelines and regulations. As healthcare regulations and coding systems evolve, coding professionals must actively pursue continuing education to ensure their practice reflects current standards.

Professional Integrity in Coding Practice

Professional integrity manifests in daily coding decisions through consistent application of coding guidelines and conventions. This includes maintaining independence in clinical judgment while collaborating effectively with healthcare providers and other stakeholders. Coding professionals must often balance multiple perspectives while adhering to established coding principles.

When encountering unclear documentation, professional integrity requires initiating appropriate queries rather than making assumptions. These queries should be constructed objectively, avoiding any leading questions that might influence provider responses. The goal remains accurate code assignment rather than achieving specific financial outcomes.

Code of Ethics for Coding Professionals

Professional coding organizations have established formal codes of ethics that provide detailed guidance for ethical practice. These codes typically address:

Professional Conduct

Maintaining high standards of personal and professional behavior that reflect positively on the profession. This includes treating colleagues, healthcare providers, and patients with respect while maintaining appropriate professional boundaries.

Table. Common Ethical Challenges and Resolution Approaches

Ethical Challenge	Description	Resolution Approach
Financial Pressure	Pressure to optimize coding for revenue	• Adhere to documented clinical facts only • Document decision rationale • Escalate to compliance officer if needed
Documentation Gaps	Unclear or incomplete documentation	• Initiate objective queries • Avoid assumptions • Request additional documentation
Conflicting Guidelines	Multiple interpretations possible	• Follow official coding guidelines • Consult coding authorities • Document decision logic
Provider Disagreements	Differences in coding interpretation	• Maintain professional communication • Present guideline evidence • Involve appropriate leadership

Confidentiality

Protecting patient information and maintaining strict compliance with privacy regulations. This extends beyond HIPAA requirements to include professional discretion in all communications about patient care.

Coding Accuracy

Striving for precision in code assignment and supporting documentation requirements. This includes reporting any identified errors and participating in correction processes.

Ethical Decision-Making Framework

When confronting ethical challenges, coding professionals should follow a structured decision-making framework. This process begins with identifying the ethical issue at hand and gathering all relevant information, including applicable coding guidelines, organizational policies, and regulatory requirements.

The framework should include consideration of multiple perspectives, potential consequences of various actions, and alignment with professional ethical standards. For complex situations, consultation with supervisors or compliance officers may be necessary to ensure appropriate resolution.

Professional Responsibility and Accountability

Coding professionals bear significant responsibility for the accuracy and integrity of healthcare claims. This responsibility includes maintaining appropriate documentation of coding decisions, participating in quality improvement activities, and reporting potential compliance concerns through appropriate channels.

Accountability extends to acknowledging and correcting errors when identified. Rather than viewing errors as failures, professional responsibility requires treating them as opportunities for improvement and learning.

Confidentiality and Privacy Considerations

Beyond regulatory compliance, ethical coding practice requires careful attention to patient privacy. This includes accessing only those records necessary for coding purposes, maintaining appropriate security measures for coding resources, and ensuring confidential handling of all patient information.

Accurate and Complete Code Assignment

Ethical coding requires complete and accurate code assignment based on available documentation. This includes assigning all relevant codes supported by documentation, not just those that affect reimbursement. Complete coding provides an accurate picture of patient care and supports quality metrics and public health data.

Ethical Documentation Practices

Documentation practices must support the integrity of the medical record. When requesting additional documentation through queries, coding professionals must maintain objectivity and avoid leading questions that might compromise the integrity of provider responses.

Conflict Resolution in Coding

When facing coding conflicts, professionals must navigate disagreements while maintaining ethical standards. This might involve conflicts between:

- Different interpretations of coding guidelines
- Pressure to maximize reimbursement versus accurate coding
- Provider documentation and coding requirements
- Organizational goals and professional ethics

Resolution should focus on maintaining coding integrity while fostering positive professional relationships. This often requires clear communication, documentation of decision-making processes, and appropriate escalation when necessary

FRAUD AND ABUSE PREVENTION

Healthcare fraud and abuse prevention represents a critical component of medical coding compliance. Understanding, identifying, and preventing fraudulent coding practices protects healthcare organizations while ensuring proper reimbursement for legitimate services.

Healthcare Fraud and Abuse

Healthcare fraud involves intentional deception or misrepresentation made to obtain unauthorized benefits. In contrast, abuse typically refers to practices that directly or indirectly result in unnecessary costs, though they may not constitute intentional deception. This distinction becomes crucial when determining appropriate responses and potential penalties.

Common Types of Coding Fraud

Several patterns of fraudulent coding practices frequently appear in healthcare settings. Understanding these patterns helps coding professionals identify and prevent potential fraud:

Upcoding represents one of the most common forms of coding fraud, occurring when providers bill for more complex services than actually rendered. For example, reporting a level 5 evaluation and management service when documentation supports only a level 3 visit constitutes upcoding.

Unbundling occurs when separate codes are reported for services that should be reported under a single comprehensive code. This practice artificially inflates reimbursement by circumventing correct coding initiatives and bundling rules.

Billing for services not rendered represents direct fraud, involving claims for procedures or services that never occurred. This might include billing for cancelled procedures or reporting services to patients who never presented for care.

Identification and Prevention Strategies

Effective fraud prevention requires a multi-layered approach combining systematic controls, education, and monitoring:

Documentation Review Protocols

Establishing robust documentation review procedures helps prevent fraudulent coding. These protocols should include:

- Verification of service delivery through multiple sources, such as nursing notes, medication administration records, and procedure notes
- Comparison of documented services against standard care protocols
- Review of timing and sequence of services for logical consistency

Monitoring Systems

Implementing comprehensive monitoring systems helps identify potential fraud patterns:

- Regular analysis of coding patterns to identify unusual trends or variations
- Tracking of claim denials and appeals to identify systematic issues
- Monitoring of individual provider coding patterns against peer benchmarks
- Review of modifier usage to ensure appropriate application

Education and Training

Ongoing education forms a crucial component of fraud prevention:

- Regular training on proper coding practices and documentation requirements
- Updates on new fraud schemes and prevention strategies
  Education about personal and organizational consequences of fraudulent practices
- Guidance on identifying and reporting suspicious activities

Compliance Program Development

A robust compliance program serves as the foundation for fraud prevention:

Written Policies and Procedures

Developing and maintaining clear policies addressing:

- Code selection criteria
- Documentation requirements
- Query processes
- Audit procedures
- Reporting mechanisms for suspected fraud

Internal Controls

Implementing effective internal controls including:

- Separation of duties in coding and billing processes
- Multiple levels of review for high-risk claims
- Documentation verification procedures
- Access controls for coding and billing systems

Response Protocols

Establishing clear procedures for responding to identified issues:

- Investigation protocols for suspected fraud

- Corrective action planning
- Self-disclosure procedures
- Documentation of resolution steps

Federal Regulations and Penalties

Understanding applicable regulations and potential penalties helps reinforce the importance of fraud prevention:

False Claims Act

The False Claims Act imposes significant penalties for knowingly submitting false claims to government healthcare programs. Penalties can include:

- Substantial monetary fines per false claim
- Treble damages
- Potential criminal prosecution
- Exclusion from federal healthcare programs

Anti-Kickback Statute

This statute prohibits offering, paying, soliciting, or receiving anything of value to induce referrals of federal healthcare program business.

Stark Law

The Stark Law restricts physician self-referral for designated health services payable by Medicare or Medicaid.

Whistleblower Protection

Organizations must establish and communicate clear whistleblower protection policies:

Confidential Reporting Mechanisms

- Anonymous hotlines
- Protected reporting channels
- Documentation of reports and responses

Non-Retaliation Policies

- Clear statements prohibiting retaliation
- Protection for good-faith reporters
- Investigation procedures for retaliation claims

Documentation and Audit Procedures

Regular auditing plays a vital role in fraud prevention:

Internal Audits

- Systematic review of coding accuracy
- Documentation compliance verification
- Pattern analysis and trending
- Focus on high-risk areas

External Audits

- Independent review of coding practices
- Validation of internal findings
- Identification of improvement opportunities

Recovery and Correction

When issues are identified, proper handling becomes crucial:

Immediate Correction

- Prompt correction of identified errors
- Implementation of preventive measures
- Documentation of corrective actions

Self-Disclosure

- Evaluation of self-disclosure requirements
- Proper notification to relevant authorities
- Implementation of corrective action plans

HIPAA COMPLIANCE

The Health Insurance Portability and Accountability Act (HIPAA) establishes national standards for the protection of individuals' medical records and other personal health information. For medical coders and healthcare organizations, HIPAA compliance represents a fundamental requirement in managing protected health information (PHI).

Privacy Rule Requirements

The HIPAA Privacy Rule establishes national standards for the protection of individuals' medical records and other personal health information. Under this rule, patients maintain specific rights regarding their health information, including the right to examine and obtain copies of their health records, request corrections to their information, and receive a notice of privacy practices. Patients can also request restrictions on certain uses and disclosures of their information and receive an accounting of disclosures.

Healthcare organizations must carefully manage the release of PHI, limiting disclosures to specific permitted purposes. These include treatment, payment, and healthcare operations purposes, uses with patient authorization, limited data sets for research, public health activities, and law enforcement purposes. Each disclosure must be evaluated against these permitted uses to ensure compliance.

Security Rule Implementation

The HIPAA Security Rule requires appropriate administrative, physical, and technical safeguards to ensure the confidentiality, integrity, and security of electronic protected health information. Administrative safeguards encompass security management processes, including risk analysis and management, information system activity review, and security incident procedures. Organizations must implement workforce security measures through proper authorization, supervision, and access management protocols.

Table. HIPAA Security Rule Implementation Matrix

Safeguard Type	Requirements	Implementation Examples
Administrative	• Security management	• Risk analysis
	• Workforce security	• Access management
	• Training programs	• Security policies
Physical	• Facility access control	• Locked areas
	• Workstation security	• Screen protectors
	• Device controls	• Equipment tracking
Technical	• Access control	• Unique user IDs
	• Audit controls	• Activity logs
	• Encryption	• Secure transmission
	• Authentication	• Password policies

Physical safeguards focus on facility access controls and workstation security. Organizations must maintain facility security plans, implement access control and validation procedures, and establish proper device and media controls. These measures protect both electronic systems and physical records containing protected health information.

Technical safeguards require implementation of access controls, including unique user identification, emergency access procedures, and automatic logoff mechanisms. Organizations must also maintain audit controls through hardware, software, and procedural mechanisms that track and examine system activities.

Protected Health Information Management

Protected Health Information includes identifiable patient data such as names, dates related to an individual, contact information, Social Security numbers, medical record numbers, and biometric identifiers. Organizations must implement the minimum necessary standard, ensuring that access to and disclosure of PHI is limited to what is required for specific purposes.

Security Incidents and Breach Notification

Organizations must maintain clear procedures for identifying and responding to potential security breaches. When breaches occur, notifications must be made without unreasonable delay, not to exceed 60 days. These notifications must include specific information about the breach, steps individuals should take to protect themselves, and measures the organization is taking to prevent future incidents.

Business Associate Relationships

Healthcare organizations must establish written agreements with business associates who handle protected health information. These agreements define responsibilities, security expectations, and breach notification obligations. Regular monitoring of business associate compliance helps ensure ongoing protection of patient information.

Training and Education Programs

Comprehensive HIPAA training forms an essential

component of compliance efforts. New employees must receive initial training covering privacy and security requirements, organization-specific policies, and individual responsibilities. Ongoing education ensures staff remain current with regulatory changes, emerging security threats, and updated organizational policies.

Documentation and Record Retention

Organizations must maintain detailed documentation of their HIPAA compliance efforts, including written privacy policies and procedures, training records, and security incident reports. These records must be retained according to federal and state requirements, organizational policies, and legal considerations.

Enforcement and Compliance Monitoring

HIPAA violations are categorized based on severity, ranging from unknowing violations to willful neglect. Penalties vary accordingly, considering factors such as the violation category, number of violations, history of compliance, and cooperation with investigations. Organizations should conduct regular compliance assessments and prepare for potential external audits through proper documentation management and staff preparation.

Maintaining HIPAA compliance requires ongoing attention to evolving regulations and emerging security threats. Through comprehensive implementation of these requirements, healthcare organizations can protect patient information while maintaining efficient operations. Regular review and updates of compliance measures ensure continued effectiveness in an evolving healthcare environment

DOCUMENTATION REQUIREMENTS

Documentation in medical coding serves as the foundation for accurate code assignment and compliant billing practices. Proper documentation supports medical necessity, justifies reimbursement, and provides a complete picture of patient care.

Medical Record Documentation Standards

Medical record documentation must be clear, consistent, and comprehensive. Documentation should reflect the patient's condition, services provided, and medical necessity for treatments. Healthcare providers must document all relevant clinical information, including patient history, physical examination findings, assessment, treatment plans, and outcomes.

Every entry in the medical record must be dated, timed, and authenticated by the responsible provider. Documentation should occur at the time of service or as soon as possible afterward to ensure accuracy. Late entries must be clearly identified as such and include the current date along with the date of the actual service.

Supporting Documentation for Code Assignment

Code assignment must be based solely on provider documentation in the medical record. Coders cannot make clinical assumptions or interpret clinical information beyond what is explicitly documented. When documentation supports multiple coding options, the documentation must clearly indicate the most specific diagnosis or procedure.

Clinical documentation should support all elements required for specific code assignment. For example, when coding complications, the record must establish a clear cause-and-effect relationship between the condition and the precipitating event or procedure. Similarly, documentation for procedures must include all components required by CPT or ICD-10-PCS guidelines.

Query Process and Protocols

When documentation lacks clarity or specificity needed for accurate coding, a formal query process becomes necessary. Queries must be constructed objectively, avoiding leading questions that might influence provider responses. Each query should:

- Identify the specific documentation issue requiring clarification
- Present the clinical indicators supporting the need for clarification
- Request additional documentation or clarification using neutral language
- Allow the provider to respond with clinically supported information

Authentication Requirements

All medical record entries require proper authentication. Electronic signatures must comply with organizational policies and regulatory requirements. Authentication includes:

Provider identification with credentials

Date and time of documentation
Method of authentication (written signature, electronic signature, or digital signature)

Amendment Procedures

When corrections to documentation become necessary, specific procedures must be followed. Original entries should never be obliterated or deleted. Instead, amendments should clearly indicate:

- The nature of the correction
- The date of the amendment

- The identity of the person making the correction
  The reason for the correction

Electronic Health Record Requirements

Electronic health records must meet specific documentation requirements while maintaining security and accessibility. Systems must include:

- Audit trails tracking all access and modifications
- Version control for amended documentation
- Security measures protecting against unauthorized access
- Backup systems ensuring data preservation
- Mechanisms for producing legible copies of records

Documentation Compliance Monitoring

Organizations must implement regular monitoring of documentation practices. This includes reviewing records for:

Completeness of Documentation

Documentation must contain all required elements supporting the services provided and billed. Missing or incomplete documentation requires prompt correction through appropriate channels.

Timeliness of Documentation

Monitor documentation completion times and implement processes to ensure timely completion of all required documentation. Establish clear expectations for documentation timeframes and follow up on delayed documentation.

Quality of Documentation

Review documentation quality focusing on clarity, specificity, and medical necessity support. Provide feedback to providers on documentation patterns requiring improvement.

Record Retention Policies

Healthcare organizations must establish and maintain clear record retention policies that address:

Storage Requirements

- Secure storage systems for both active and archived records
  Protection of confidential information
- Accessibility for authorized users

Retention Periods

- Compliance with state and federal retention requirements
  Consideration of specialized retention needs
- Documentation of destruction procedures

Legal Considerations

Protection of records involved in litigation Maintenance of records for ongoing care Response to record requests and subpoenas

Ongoing Education and Training

Maintain regular education programs addressing:

- Documentation Requirements
- Updates to documentation standards
- Common documentation deficiencies
- Best practices for documentation

Compliance Issues

- Regulatory changes affecting documentation
- Audit findings and corrective actions
- Documentation improvement strategies

Quality Improvement Initiatives

Implement continuous quality improvement programs focusing on documentation:

Regular Assessment

- Review documentation patterns and identify areas for improvement
- Track documentation deficiencies and trends
- Measure improvement over time

Feedback Mechanisms

- Provide constructive feedback to providers
- Share best practices and success stories
- Address documentation challenges promptly

Corrective Action Planning

- Develop targeted improvement plans
- Monitor effectiveness of interventions
- Adjust approaches based on outcomes

QUALITY ASSURANCE

Quality assurance in medical coding encompasses systematic monitoring and evaluation of coding accuracy, consistency, and compliance. An effective quality assurance program ensures high-quality coding output while identifying areas for improvement and educational needs.

Components of Quality Assurance Programs

A comprehensive quality assurance program incorporates multiple elements working together to maintain coding quality. At its core, the program must establish clear quality metrics, implement regular monitoring processes, and provide mechanisms for continuous improvement. These components work together to create a culture of quality throughout the coding operation.

Table. Quality Assurance Performance Metrics

Metric Category	Measurement Criteria	Target Range
Accuracy	• Diagnosis code accuracy	95-98%
	• Procedure code accuracy	95-98%
	• Modifier usage	95-98%
Productivity	• Records per hour	Based on case type: • Inpatient: 2-3/hr • Outpatient: 4-6/hr
Documentation	• Query response rate	>85%
	• Query quality	>90%
	• Timeliness	48-72 hours
Compliance	• Critical error rate	<2%
	• Denial rate	<5%
	• Appeal success	>75%

Quality Review Process

The review process begins with establishing baseline accuracy requirements and determining appropriate sample sizes for review. Reviews should examine code assignment accuracy, supporting documentation, and compliance with coding guidelines. Each review must evaluate both technical accuracy and the coder's interpretation of clinical documentation.

Sample selection should incorporate both random and focused reviews. While random sampling provides insight into overall quality levels, focused reviews target high-risk areas, new procedures, or areas where previous issues have been identified. The combination ensures comprehensive quality monitoring while efficiently utilizing review resources.

Performance Metrics and Standards

Organizations must establish clear performance standards for coding accuracy. These standards typically address accuracy rates for diagnosis coding, procedure coding, and modifier usage. Standards should consider complexity levels and differentiate between critical and non-critical errors.

Beyond simple accuracy rates, quality metrics should evaluate:

- Productivity levels balanced against accuracy
- Query rates and quality
- Documentation improvement suggestions
- Compliance with internal policies
- Timeliness of coding completion

Error Analysis and Trending

When errors are identified, thorough analysis helps determine root causes and appropriate corrective actions. Error analysis should examine patterns in:

Error types and frequency

- Documentation issues contributing to errors
- Specific procedures or diagnoses involved
- Individual coder performance patterns
- Systemic issues affecting multiple coders

Educational Support and Development

Quality assurance findings should drive educational initiatives. When trends indicate specific knowledge gaps or areas of confusion, targeted education can address these issues effectively. Education may include:

- Individual mentoring for specific challenges
- Group training on common error patterns
- Updates on coding guideline changes

- Review of complex coding scenarios
- Sharing of best practices and lessons learned

Monitoring and Feedback Systems

Regular monitoring ensures sustained quality improvement. Feedback systems should provide timely information to both coders and management regarding quality performance. This feedback helps maintain accountability while identifying areas requiring additional support or intervention.

Corrective Action Planning

When quality issues are identified, structured corrective action plans help ensure effective resolution. These plans should:

- Define specific performance issues
- Establish clear improvement goals
- Outline required actions and timelines
- Provide necessary resources and support
- Monitor progress toward goals

Documentation of Quality Activities

Maintain comprehensive documentation of all quality assurance activities, including:

- Review findings and trends
- Educational interventions
- Corrective actions taken
- Progress monitoring results
- Overall program effectiveness

Continuous Program Improvement

Quality assurance programs must evolve to address changing needs and requirements. Regular evaluation of program effectiveness helps identify opportunities for improvement in:

- Review methodologies
- Performance metrics
- Educational approaches
- Feedback mechanisms
- Resource allocation

External Quality Requirements

Consider requirements from external entities such as:

- Regulatory compliance standards
- Accreditation requirements
- Payer-specific quality programs
- Industry best practices
- Professional certification standards

Technology Integration

Utilize appropriate technology tools to support quality assurance efforts. These tools may include:

- Coding audit software
- Performance tracking systems
- Educational platforms
- Documentation analysis tools
- Report generation systems

Team Collaboration

Foster collaboration between quality assurance staff, coders, and clinical documentation specialists. This collaboration helps ensure comprehensive quality improvement and supports consistent application of coding guidelines.

Success Measurement

Establish clear measures for program success, including:

- Accuracy rate improvements
- Reduction in denial rates

- Enhanced documentation quality
- Improved productivity metrics
- Decreased error patterns

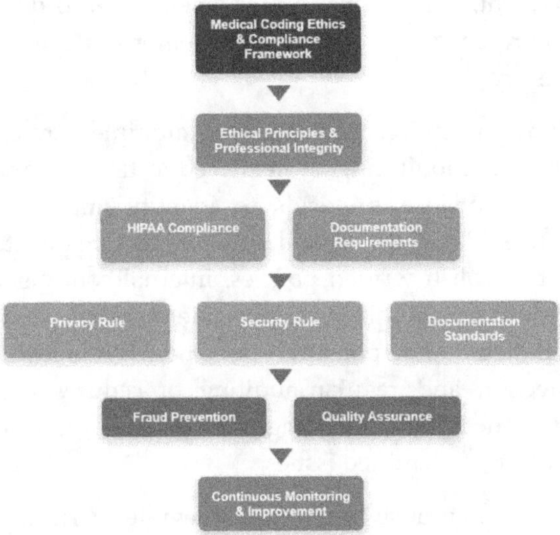

Summary

Medical coding practices demand strict adherence to ethical principles, regulatory compliance, and comprehensive documentation standards to maintain healthcare revenue integrity. The foundation rests on truthful and accurate code assignment based solely on clinical documentation, regardless of financial implications. Professional integrity requires current knowledge of coding guidelines, appropriate query processes, and collaboration with healthcare providers while maintaining independence in clinical judgment.

HIPAA compliance establishes essential frameworks for protecting patient health information through privacy rules, security measures, and breach notification protocols. Healthcare organizations must implement administrative, physical, and technical safeguards while maintaining business associate agreements and comprehensive training programs. Documentation requirements emphasize clear, consistent, and authenticated medical records that support code assignment and demonstrate medical necessity.

Fraud prevention encompasses multiple strategies, including monitoring systems, education programs, and compliance protocols to identify and prevent practices like upcoding and unbundling. Organizations must establish written policies, internal controls, and response protocols while understanding federal regulations and potential penalties. Whistleblower protection and regular auditing procedures ensure systematic review of coding practices and appropriate handling of identified issues.

Quality assurance programs integrate performance metrics, error analysis, and educational support to maintain high coding standards. Regular monitoring and feedback systems help identify areas for improvement while supporting continuous program development. The framework emphasizes team collaboration, technology integration, and success measurements to ensure sustained quality in coding operations.

Multiple Choice Questions

1. Which principle serves as the primary foundation of coding ethics?
   a) Financial optimization
   b) Truthfulness
   c) Speed
   d) Flexibility

2. When documentation supports multiple interpretations, coders should:
   a) Choose the most financially beneficial option
   b) Select the most clinically appropriate option
   c) Ask another coder for their preference
   d) Leave it uncoded

3. A query to a healthcare provider should be:
   a) Leading to achieve desired response
   b) Objective and unbiased
   c) Focused on financial outcomes
   d) Informal and casual

4. Which is NOT a common type of coding fraud?
   a) Upcoding
   b) Unbundling
   c) Documentation improvement
   d) Billing for services not rendered

5. The HIPAA Privacy Rule gives patients the right to:
   a) Change their provider's documentation
   b) Access their health records
   c) Modify billing codes
   d) Choose their insurance provider

6. Under HIPAA, a breach notification must be made within:
   a) 30 days
   b) 45 days
   c) 60 days
   d) 90 days

7. Medical record documentation must be:
   a) Clear, consistent, and comprehensive
   b) Brief and general
   c) Focused only on billing requirements
   d) Written in technical language

8. When making corrections to documentation, one should:
   a) Delete the original entry
   b) Use white-out
   c) Clearly indicate the nature and date of correction
   d) Make changes without notation

9. Which is a proper component of a quality assurance program?
   a) Random sampling only
   b) Annual reviews only
   c) Both random and focused reviews
   d) Informal peer review

10. Professional integrity in coding requires:
    a) Maximizing reimbursement
    b) Maintaining current knowledge
    c) Avoiding queries
    d) Working independently only

11. The False Claims Act penalties can include:
    a) Verbal warnings only
    b) Treble damages
    c) Simple fines
    d) Temporary suspension

12. Protected Health Information (PHI) includes:
    a) Only medical diagnoses
    b) Only insurance information
    c) Only contact details
    d) Names, dates, contact information, and identifiers

13. In electronic health records, which is required?
    a) Audit trails
    b) Manual backup only
    c) Limited access controls
    d) Weekly system shutdown

14. Quality assurance feedback should be:
    a) Annual only
    b) Timely and specific
    c) General and vague
    d) Focused only on errors

15. Business Associate Agreements are required for:
    a) All hospital employees
    b) Patients only
    c) Entities handling PHI
    d) Insurance companies only

16. Documentation authentication requires:
    a) Provider identification only
    b) Date only

c) Provider ID, date, time, and method
d) Electronic signature only

17. When facing coding conflicts, professionals should:
a) Always agree with management
b) Maintain coding integrity while fostering relationships
c) Ignore organizational policies
d) Avoid documentation

18. The minimum necessary standard under HIPAA refers to:
a) Minimum staffing requirements
b) Limiting PHI access and disclosure
c) Minimum documentation requirements
d) Basic security measures

19. Quality assurance error analysis should examine:
a) Only critical errors
b) Individual performance only
c) Patterns and trends in all errors
d) Random samples only

20. Proper query construction should:
a) Lead to desired responses
b) Focus on financial outcomes
c) Present clinical indicators objectively
d) Be informal

21. Recovery and correction procedures require:
a) Immediate correction of identified errors
b) Waiting for annual review

c) Informal correction processes
d) Verbal agreements only

22. Technical safeguards under HIPAA include:
a) Building security only
b) Unique user identification and access controls
c) Paper record storage
d) Staff training only

23. Documentation compliance monitoring should review:
a) Completeness only
b) Timeliness only
c) Quality only
d) Completeness, timeliness, and quality

24. Coding professionals must maintain:
a) Financial goals only
b) Production speed only
c) Professional boundaries and confidentiality
d) Personal relationships with providers

25. Quality assurance success measurements should include:
a) Financial metrics only
b) Productivity only
c) Multiple metrics including accuracy and denial rates
d) Staff satisfaction only

List of Important Questions

1. Define coding ethics and explain its fundamental principles in healthcare revenue management.
2. How do professional integrity and ethical decision-making frameworks influence daily coding practices?
3. Describe the common types of coding fraud and outline prevention strategies.
4. What are the key components of a comprehensive HIPAA compliance program?
5. Explain the Privacy and Security Rule requirements under HIPAA.
6. Discuss the importance of documentation standards in medical coding.
7. What constitutes proper authentication and amendment procedures in medical records?
8. How does a query process support accurate code assignment?
9. Outline the components of an effective quality assurance program in medical coding.
10. Describe the role of performance metrics and standards in maintaining coding quality.
11. What are the essential elements of fraud and abuse prevention strategies?
12. Explain the significance of business associate agreements in HIPAA compliance.
13. How do documentation requirements support medical necessity and reimbursement?
14. Describe the process for handling security incidents and breach notifications.
15. What are the key considerations in developing and maintaining record retention policies?
16. How do continuous quality improvement initiatives enhance coding accuracy?
17. Explain the importance of error analysis and trending in quality assurance.

18. What role does technology play in supporting coding compliance and quality?
19. Describe the components of a comprehensive coding education and training program.
20. How do federal regulations impact coding practices and compliance programs?

Bibliography

1. Manchikanti L, Helm S, Benyamin RM, Hirsch JA. Merit-Based Incentive Payment System: Meaningful Changes in the Final Rule. Pain Physician. 2017;20(1):1-12.
2. Bowman S. Impact of Electronic Health Record Systems on Information Integrity: Quality and Safety Implications. Perspect Health Inf Manag. 2013;10(Fall):1c.
3. O'Malley KJ, Cook KF, Price MD, et al. Measuring Diagnoses: ICD Code Accuracy. Health Serv Res. 2005;40(5 Pt 2):1620-1639.
4. Cohen GR, Friedman CP, Ryan AM, et al. Variation in Physicians' Electronic Health Record Documentation and Potential Patient Harm from That Variation. J Gen Intern Med. 2019;34(11):2355-2367.
5. Cassidy BS. Maintaining Ethical Standards in the Coding Process. J AHIMA. 2011;82(4):42-44.
6. Price-Haywood EG, Luo Q, Monlezun D. Impact of Healthcare Information Technology on Clinical Quality. Ochsner J. 2019;19(2):143-151.
7. Abdelhak M, Grostick S, Hanken MA. Health Information: Management of a Strategic Resource. 5th ed. St. Louis: Elsevier; 2016.
8. Butler M. Managing the Risks of Copy and Paste in EHRs. J AHIMA. 2015;86(7):24-27.
9. Blumenthal D, Tavenner M. The "Meaningful Use" Regulation for Electronic Health Records. N Engl J Med. 2010;363(6):501-504.
10. Stanfill MH, Williams M. Clinical Documentation Integrity: Best Practices for Healthcare Organizations. J AHIMA. 2017;88(7):32-37.
11. Russo R. Documentation and Data Improvement Fundamentals. J AHIMA. 2004;75(7):42-45.
12. Dimick C. Documentation Bad Habits: Shortcuts in

Electronic Records Pose Risk. J AHIMA. 2008;79(6):40-43.

13. Weiner MG, Embi PJ. Toward Reuse of Clinical Data for Research and Quality Improvement: The End of the Beginning? Ann Intern Med. 2009;151(5):359-360.
14. Houser SH, Meadows JW. Transitioning to Electronic Health Records: Key Factors for Success. J AHIMA. 2007;78(9):69-73.
15. Dimick C. Quality Check: An Overview of Quality Measures and Their Uses. J AHIMA. 2010;81(9):34-38.
16. Giannangelo K, Hyde L. Documentation Detective: Seven Steps to CDI Success. J AHIMA. 2010;81(1):46-50.
17. Rode D. Embracing ICD-10 Advocacy: HIM Professionals Must Involve Physicians, Build Alliances to Reach Goals. J AHIMA. 2010;81(2):24-28.
18. Murphy B, Waters R. The Role of Healthcare Internal Auditors in EHR Implementation. J AHIMA. 2012;83(4):46-50.
19. Watzlaf VJ, Zeng X, Jarymowycz C, Firouzan PA. Standards for the Content of the Electronic Health Record. Perspect Health Inf Manag. 2004;1:1.
20. Wilson JF. Health Insurance Portability and Accountability Act Privacy Rule Causes Ongoing Concerns among Clinicians and Researchers. Ann Intern Med. 2006;145(4):313-316.

CHAPTER 12

CPC EXAM STRATEGIES AND CASE STUDIES

Author

Mr. Vijay Chauhan, Assistant Professor, School of Pharmaceutical Sciences, Atmiya University, Rajkot, Gujarat, India

Abstract

Comprehensive guidance for success in the CPC examination, focusing on essential strategies across multiple domains. The examination, consisting of 150 multiple-choice questions completed in 5 hours and 40 minutes, requires efficient time management, allocating approximately 2.25 minutes per question. Strategic approaches include dividing the exam into manageable segments, organizing reference materials, and implementing systematic question analysis methods. Question analysis emphasizes identifying key clinical information, proper documentation review, and accurate code selection. The process of elimination technique helps evaluate multiple-choice options methodically, comparing code components and verifying selections through index and tabular reviews. Common pitfalls encompass misreading questions, documentation interpretation errors, and guideline application mistakes. Test-taking strategies emphasize proper preparation, anxiety management, and strategic answering techniques. The guidance includes practical tips for exam day success, focusing on time management, physical comfort, material organization, and maintaining focus. Emergency strategies address time management issues and anxiety control, ensuring examinees can complete all questions effectively while maintaining accuracy.

Keywords: *Time management; Medical coding examination; Clinical documentation analysis; Code selection methodology; Test-taking strategies*

Learning Objectives

After completion of the chapter, the learner should be able to:

- Develop and implement effective time management strategies for completing 150 questions within the allocated examination time.
- Apply systematic methods for analyzing clinical scenarios and selecting appropriate medical codes using reference materials efficiently.
- Identify and avoid common examination pitfalls through proper documentation interpretation and accurate guideline application.
- Utilize the process of elimination technique effectively to evaluate multiple-choice options and verify code selections.
- Implement comprehensive test-taking strategies, including preparation methods, anxiety management techniques, and systematic review processes.
- Master practical exam day techniques for maintaining focus, managing materials, and addressing time management challenges.

TIME MANAGEMENT TECHNIQUES

The CPC examination is a comprehensive test consisting of 150 multiple-choice questions that must be completed within 5 hours and 40 minutes. Understanding the exam structure and developing effective time management is crucial for success. This timing allows approximately 2.25 minutes per question, making efficient time usage essential.

Exam Format Overview

The examination is divided into several sections covering various aspects of medical coding, including surgical procedures, medical concepts, and coding guidelines. Each question presents a clinical scenario or coding challenge that requires careful analysis. The questions are not arranged by difficulty level or subject matter, requiring examinees to adapt their approach throughout the test.

Time Distribution

The 5-hour and 40-minute duration includes the total testing period from start to finish. This time must accommodate:

- Reading and analyzing clinical scenarios
- Reviewing multiple code options
- Consulting coding manuals and guidelines
- Marking answers on the answer sheet
- Periodic progress checks
- Final review if time permits

Strategic Time Planning

Successful candidates typically divide the exam into manageable segments. A practical approach is to divide the exam into three sections of 50 questions each, allocating roughly 1 hour and 50 minutes per section. This division allows for structured progress monitoring and helps maintain a steady pace throughout the examination.

Initial Assessment Period

The first 15-20 minutes of the exam are crucial for:

- Understanding the exam layout
- Reviewing general instructions
- Organizing reference materials
- Establishing a comfortable working setup

- Planning question-answering strategy

Progress Monitoring

Regular time checks are essential but should not become a source of anxiety. Establish specific checkpoints, such as:

- First hour: Complete approximately 25-30 questions
- Midpoint (2 hours, 50 minutes): Complete 75 questions
- Final hour: Complete remaining questions and review

Table. Recommended Time Management Breakdown

Time Period	Target Completion	Activities
First 15-20 minutes	Setup and Organization	• Review instructions • Organize materials • Plan strategy
First 1 hour, 50 minutes	50 questions	• Complete first section • Basic progress check
Second 1 hour, 50 minutes	100 questions (cumulative)	• Complete second section • Midpoint evaluation
Final 1 hour, 50 minutes	All 150 questions	• Complete final section • Review marked questions
Last 20 minutes	Final Review	• Verify all answers • Check completion

Adjustment Considerations

The examination structure requires flexibility in time management. Some questions will require more time due to:

- Complex clinical scenarios
- Multiple procedure codes
- Detailed documentation review

Guideline verification requirements

Different types of questions demand varying amounts of time. While some straightforward questions might take less than a minute, complex surgical scenarios could require several minutes of analysis. Understanding this variability helps in allocating time appropriately during the examination.

Reference Material Organization

Efficient time management relies heavily on organized reference materials. Before the exam:

- Arrange coding manuals for quick access
- Tab frequently used sections
- Familiarize yourself with manual layouts
- Practice locating information quickly

Time Management Tools

The examination allows basic timing devices. Utilize:

- A simple watch or timer
- Progress tracking methods
- Time management worksheets
- Systematic marking systems

Emergency Time Strategies

If falling behind schedule:

- Focus on questions you can answer quickly
- Mark complex questions for later review
- Maintain awareness of remaining time
- Adjust pace as needed without rushing

QUESTION ANALYSIS METHODS

CPC exam questions typically fall into several distinct categories, each requiring a specific approach. Straightforward coding questions require direct code lookup and selection, while complex scenarios demand thorough analysis of multiple elements. Some questions focus on specific coding guidelines or documentation requirements.

Common question types include:

- Single procedure coding
- Multiple procedure scenarios
- Diagnosis code selection
- Modifier application
- Compliance and guidelines

Table. Question Type Analysis Guide

Question Type	**Features**	**Time Allocation**	**Special Considerations**
Single Procedure	• One primary code • Direct lookup	1-2 minutes	• Verify anatomical site • Check modifiers
Multiple Procedures	• Multiple codes • Bundling rules	2-3 minutes	• Check sequencing • Review guidelines
Diagnosis Selection	• ICD-10 codes • Clinical indicators	2 minutes	• Specificity level • Supporting documentation
Compliance/Guide	• Rule	2-3	• Current

Question Type	Features	Time Allocation	Special Considerations
lines	interpretation • Policy application	minutes	guidelines • Documentation requirements
Documentation Analysis	• Complex scenarios • Multiple elements	3+ minutes	• Complete review • Link all elements

Documentation requirements

B. Identifying Key Information

Critical information appears throughout question scenarios. Effective analysis requires identifying essential elements while filtering out less relevant details. Key information typically includes:

Patient Demographics

Age, gender, and other relevant patient characteristics that may affect code selection or indicate specific conditions.

Clinical Indicators

Signs, symptoms, and diagnostic findings that support diagnosis code selection and medical necessity.

Procedural Details

Specific techniques, approaches, and anatomical locations that determine procedure code selection.

Time Elements

Dates of service, timing of procedures, and follow-up periods that affect code selection and modifier usage.

C. Clinical Scenario Analysis

Successful clinical scenario analysis requires a systematic approach:

Initial Review

Read the entire scenario carefully to understand the overall clinical picture before attempting to select codes.

Component Identification

Break down complex scenarios into individual billable components, identifying each distinct service or procedure.

Medical Necessity Evaluation

Assess whether documented findings support the procedures performed and diagnoses coded.

Sequencing Determination

Establish the appropriate order for multiple procedures and diagnoses based on coding guidelines.

D. Code Selection Approach

Code selection follows a methodical process to ensure accuracy:

Preliminary Code Location

Use the index to locate potential codes based on key terms from the clinical scenario.

Verification Process

Review code descriptions in the tabular list to confirm the most specific code selection.

Guideline Application

Apply relevant coding guidelines, including procedure-specific rules and diagnosis coding conventions.

Modifier Consideration

Evaluate the need for modifiers based on the clinical scenario and documentation provided.

E. Documentation Review Skills

Documentation review requires attention to specific elements:

Essential Components

Verify that documentation includes all required elements for the codes being considered.

Supporting Information

Ensure clinical documentation supports the specificity level of selected codes.

Completeness Assessment

Check that all relevant aspects of the service are documented sufficiently.

Linking Elements

Confirm clear connections between diagnoses and procedures in the documentation.

Common Documentation Patterns

Recognize standard documentation formats and required elements for different service types.

Documentation Deficiencies

Identify when documentation lacks necessary elements for code assignment.

Successful question analysis combines these elements into a cohesive approach:

Strategic Reading

Develop efficient methods for identifying relevant information while maintaining accuracy.

Pattern Recognition

Learn to recognize common question formats and typical clinical scenarios.

Critical Thinking

Apply coding knowledge and guidelines to resolve complex coding situations.

Decision Making

Make informed choices based on available information and coding guidelines.

Time Management

Balance thorough analysis with efficient processing to complete all questions within the time limit.

Through consistent practice with these methods, candidates develop the analytical skills necessary for successful completion of the CPC examination. Regular application of these techniques during exam preparation helps establish effective habits for actual exam conditions.

Remember that question analysis is not just about finding the right answer but understanding why that answer is correct

PROCESS OF ELIMINATION

A. Systematic Approach to Options

The process of elimination in CPC exam questions requires a methodical approach to evaluate multiple-choice options. This systematic method helps identify the most accurate code selection while ruling out incorrect options.

Begin by examining each option without immediately selecting an answer. Compare the given options against the clinical scenario and documentation, noting key differences between similar codes. Consider code components such as anatomical sites, approaches, and additional descriptors that distinguish between options.

Work through options sequentially, marking clearly incorrect choices first. This narrows the field of possible answers and allows focused attention on more viable options. Document brief notes about why specific options are eliminated to prevent second-guessing during review.

B. Identifying Clearly Incorrect Choices

Some options can be eliminated quickly based on obvious mismatches with the clinical scenario. Common reasons for immediate elimination include:

Anatomical Site Mismatch

When the anatomical location in the code description doesn't match the documented site of service.

Wrong Procedure Type

Codes describing fundamentally different procedures than what was documented in the scenario.

Invalid Code Combinations

Options that would create inappropriate or impossible code combinations in actual billing situations.

Outdated or Invalid Codes

Codes that are no longer valid for the date of service or aren't appropriate for the setting.

C. Comparing Similar Code Options

After eliminating obviously incorrect choices, careful comparison of remaining options becomes crucial:

Specificity Levels

Compare the level of detail in each code description against the documented information.

Code Components

Analyze individual components of similar codes,

including:

- Approach methods
- Device usage
- Additional procedures included
- Qualifying circumstances

Guideline Application

Review relevant coding guidelines that might affect the selection between similar codes.

D. Verification Techniques

Before making a final selection, verify remaining options through several steps:

Index Verification

Double-check index entries for key terms to ensure no better options exist.

Tabular Review

Review complete code descriptions in the tabular list for remaining options.

Guideline Confirmation

Verify that the selected code aligns with all applicable coding guidelines.

Documentation Match

Confirm the selected code matches all documented elements of the service.

E. Final Selection Methods

Make the final code selection using a confirmation process:

Positive Verification

Confirm that the selected code matches all aspects of the documented service.

Negative Verification

Verify that eliminated options contain elements that definitely exclude them from consideration.

Cross-Reference Check

Review related codes and guidelines to ensure the best possible selection.

Practical Application Tips

Time Management

Balance thorough analysis with efficient decision-making:

- Set time limits for initial option review
- Move forward if stuck between options
- Mark questions for review if needed

Common Patterns

Recognize frequent patterns in option presentation:

- Similar codes with varying specificity
- Related procedures with different approaches
- Codes with subtle differences in descriptions

Error Prevention

Avoid common mistakes in the elimination process:

- Don't eliminate options based on assumptions
- Consider all documentation before ruling out choices
- Review guidelines when uncertain

Documentation Support

Use available documentation effectively:

- Match documented elements to code descriptions
- Verify all required components are present
- Consider documentation quality and completeness

Final Verification Steps

Before moving to the next question:

- Confirm the selected answer meets all requirements
- Verify eliminated options remain invalid
- Note any uncertainties for later review
- Mark clearly eliminated options to prevent confusion during review

COMMON EXAM PITFALLS

A. Misreading Questions

Question Interpretation Errors

Examinees often fall into the trap of misinterpreting question requirements through hasty reading or assumptions. Common misreading errors include:

Missing Key Details

Overlooking critical information embedded within clinical scenarios, such as:

- Secondary procedures performed
- Specific anatomical locations
- Time elements affecting code selection
- Important modifying factors

Assumption-Based Errors

Making clinical assumptions beyond the information provided in the scenario. Successful exam completion requires working strictly with the documented information.

Context Misinterpretation

Failing to recognize the specific context of procedures or diagnoses, leading to incorrect code selection or modifier application.

B. Documentation Interpretation Errors

Clinical Documentation Analysis

Table. Common Pitfalls and Prevention Strategies

Pitfall Category	Common Errors	Prevention Strategies	Impact on Success
Time Management	• Spending too long on difficult questions • Poor progress monitoring	• Set strict time limits • Use checkpoint system	High
Documentation Review	• Missing key elements • Over-interpretation	• Systematic review process • Stick to stated facts	Critical
Code Selection	• Wrong specificity level • Incorrect anatomical site	• Double-check codes • Verify all components	High
Guideline Application	• Missing relevant guidelines • Incorrect modifier use	• Review guidelines first • Verify requirements	Critical
Answer Sheet Completion	• Skipped questions • Incorrect marking	• Regular verification • Systematic review	Moderate

Errors in documentation interpretation can significantly impact code selection:

Incomplete Review

Failing to consider all aspects of the documented service before selecting codes.

Over-interpretation

Reading more into the documentation than what is actually stated, leading to overcoding or incorrect specificity levels.

Missing Documentation Links

Failing to recognize connections between different elements of the documentation that affect code selection.

C. Guideline Application Mistakes

Common Guidelines Errors

Mistakes in applying coding guidelines often occur in several key areas:

Sequencing Errors

Incorrect application of sequencing rules for multiple procedures or diagnoses.

Modifier Misuse

Improper application or omission of required modifiers based on documented circumstances.

Bundling/Unbundling Errors

Failure to recognize when procedures are included in other services or when separate coding is appropriate.

D. Timing Issues

Time Management Problems

Poor time management can lead to various issues:

- Rushing Through Questions
- Making careless errors due to trying to maintain pace or catch up on time.
- Spending Too Much Time

- Getting stuck on difficult questions and losing time needed for other sections.
- Inadequate Review Time
- Failing to leave sufficient time for reviewing marked questions or double-checking answers.

E. Common Coding Errors

Technical Coding Mistakes

Specific coding errors that frequently appear:

- Specificity Level Errors
- Selecting codes that are either too specific or too general based on documentation.
- Anatomical Site Confusion
- Mixing up similar anatomical locations or failing to identify precise locations.
- Procedure Code Mismatches
- Selecting codes that don't exactly match the documented procedure components.

Prevention Strategies

Systematic Question Approach

Develop a consistent method for approaching each question:

- Read the entire question before consulting code books
- Identify all key elements before code selection
- Verify code choices against documentation
- Review modifiers and guidelines before finalizing

Documentation Review Process

Establish a thorough documentation review process:

- Identify all billable services
- Confirm documentation supports code specificity
- Verify medical necessity elements

- Check for required documentation components

Time Management Solutions

Implement effective time management strategies:

- Set specific time limits for each question
- Use marking system for difficult questions
- Plan regular progress checks
- Reserve adequate review time

Guideline Verification

Maintain proper guideline application:

- Review relevant guidelines before final code selection
- Verify modifier requirements
- Check bundling rules and coding conventions
- Confirm proper sequencing

Quality Control Measures

Implement personal quality checks:

- Double-check calculations and numbers
- Verify anatomical locations
- Confirm all question components are addressed
- Review marked questions systematically

Practice Techniques

Develop effective practice habits:

- Work with timed practice tests
- Review missed questions thoroughly
- Study common error patterns
- Practice with various question types

TEST-TAKING STRATEGIES

A. Preparation and Organization

Pre-Exam Organization

Proper organization sets the foundation for exam

success:

- Manual Preparation
- Tab coding manuals systematically by sections
- Mark frequently used guidelines
- Create quick-reference notes within allowed guidelines
- Ensure all materials meet exam requirements

Physical Preparation

- Get adequate rest before exam day
- Plan arrival time accounting for check-in procedures
- Prepare comfortable clothing suitable for long testing periods
- Organize required materials the night before

B. Managing Test Anxiety

Anxiety Management Techniques

Implement effective stress-reduction strategies:

- Breathing Exercises
- Practice controlled breathing during difficult questions
- Use brief relaxation techniques between sections
- Maintain steady pacing through anxiety moments

Mental Preparation

- Develop positive self-talk strategies
- Focus on preparation rather than outcomes
- Use visualization techniques for success
- Break the exam into manageable segments

C. Strategic Answering Techniques

Effective Response Methods

Develop systematic approaches to question-answering:

Initial Reading Strategy

- Read the entire question before looking at answer choices
- Identify key words and clinical indicators
- Note specific requirements or limitations
- Understand what the question is actually asking

Answer Selection Process

- Consider all options before selecting final answer
- Mark questions requiring additional review
- Use process of elimination effectively
- Trust initial instincts while verifying choices

D. Review and Double-Check Methods

Systematic Review Process

Implement thorough review procedures:

During the Exam

- Mark questions needing review
- Note uncertain answers for later verification
- Track time while reviewing marked questions
- Verify all answers are properly marked

Final Review Strategy

- Check for skipped questions
- Review marked questions systematically
- Verify answer sheet completion
- Ensure proper answer bubble filling

E. Practical Tips for Exam Day

Essential Exam Strategies

Implement proven success techniques:

Time Management

- Begin with easier questions to build confidence
- Maintain steady pacing throughout
- Allow time for breaks when needed

- Reserve adequate review time

Physical Comfort

- Take allowed breaks strategically
- Maintain good posture
- Stay hydrated
- Use stretching exercises during breaks

Material Management

- Organize reference materials efficiently
- Keep essential resources easily accessible
- Maintain clean workspace
- Use allowable markers or tabs effectively

Focus Maintenance

- Minimize distractions
- Concentrate on one question at a time
- Stay within current section
- Avoid comparing progress with others

Specific Test-Taking Tactics

Question Approach

- Read questions carefully without rushing
- Identify key words and requirements
- Consider all options before selection
- Use available scratch paper effectively

Answer Selection

- Apply systematic elimination process
- Mark uncertain answers for review
- Trust preparation and knowledge
- Avoid changing answers without clear reason

Time Optimization

- Monitor progress regularly
- Adjust pace as needed
- Use remaining time effectively

- Complete all questions, even if guessing

Error Prevention

- Double-check code selections
- Verify modifier applications
- Confirm answer sheet accuracy
- Review marked questions thoroughly

Emergency Strategies

Time Management Issues

- Skip difficult questions temporarily
- Mark questions for later review
- Maintain awareness of remaining time
- Make educated guesses if necessary

Anxiety Management

- Take deep breaths
- Focus on current question only
- Use positive self-talk
- Remember preparation efforts

Last-*Minute Checks*

- Verify all questions answered
- Check answer sheet completion
- Review marked questions
- Ensure proper identification completed

Success Mindset

- Maintain confidence in preparation
- Focus on process rather than outcome
- Use anxiety as motivation
- Trust in knowledge and abilities.

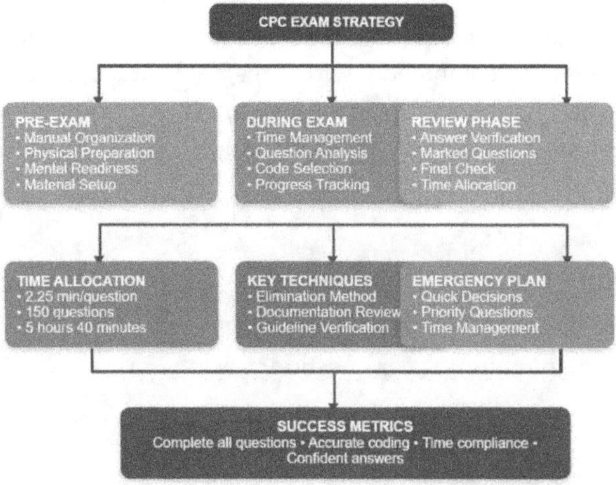

Summary

Successful completion of the CPC examination demands mastery of multiple strategic elements. Time management serves as a foundational skill, requiring examinees to efficiently navigate 150 questions within the 5-hour and 40-minute timeframe. Systematic question analysis methods, combined with organized reference materials and effective code selection techniques, form the core approach to exam success. Understanding common pitfalls, including documentation interpretation errors and guideline application mistakes, helps prevent critical errors during the examination. The process of elimination technique provides a structured method for evaluating multiple-choice options and arriving at accurate code selections. Test-taking strategies encompass proper preparation, anxiety management, and systematic review processes, while practical exam day techniques focus on maintaining physical comfort, managing materials effectively, and implementing emergency strategies when needed. The integration of these elements, combined with regular practice and thorough preparation, positions candidates for optimal performance on the CPC examination.

Multiple Choice Questions

1. The CPC examination allows approximately how many minutes per question?
   a) 1.5 minutes
   b) 2 minutes
   c) 2.25 minutes
   d) 3 minutes

2. During initial assessment, how much time should be allocated for understanding exam layout and organizing materials?
   a) 5-10 minutes
   b) 15-20 minutes
   c) 25-30 minutes
   d) 30-35 minutes

3. By the midpoint of the exam (2 hours, 50 minutes), how many questions should ideally be completed?
   a) 50 questions
   b) 65 questions
   c) 75 questions
   d) 85 questions

4. What is the recommended approach for dividing the exam questions?
   a) Two sections of 75 questions
   b) Four sections of 37-38 questions

c) Three sections of 50 questions
d) Five sections of 30 questions

5. When falling behind schedule, which strategy is most appropriate?
a) Skip all remaining questions
b) Focus on questions you can answer quickly
c) Spend more time on complex questions
d) Ignore time management completely

6. Which is NOT a key element in documentation review?
a) Essential components
b) Supporting information
c) Personal opinions
d) Linking elements

7. During the process of elimination, what should be done first?
a) Mark clearly incorrect choices
b) Select the final answer immediately
c) Skip to the next question
d) Review the guidelines

8. What is a common timing error during the examination?
a) Taking too many breaks
b) Spending excessive time on difficult questions
c) Reading too quickly
d) Using multiple timers

9. What is the total duration of the CPC examination?
a) 5 hours
b) 5 hours and 20 minutes

c) 5 hours and 40 minutes
d) 6 hours

10. Which approach is recommended for clinical scenario analysis?
a) Skip the scenario and look at codes
b) Read only the last sentence
c) Initial complete review followed by component identification
d) Random code selection

11. When should examinees verify answer sheet completion?
a) Only at the end
b) Never
c) Periodically throughout and during final review
d) Only during breaks

12. What is the best approach for managing test anxiety?
a) Ignore it completely
b) Leave the examination room
c) Practice controlled breathing techniques
d) Rush through questions

13. In documentation review, what should be verified first?
a) Modifier usage
b) Essential components
c) ICD-10 guidelines
d) CPT guidelines

14. How should reference materials be organized?
a) Randomly
b) Alphabetically only

c) By frequency of use and systematic tabbing
d) No organization needed

15. What is the recommended strategy for complex questions?
a) Skip them entirely
b) Mark for later review
c) Guess immediately
d) Spend unlimited time

16. During final review, what should be prioritized?
a) Unmarked questions only
b) Marked questions for review
c) Skipped questions only
d) Random questions

17. What is the best approach for timing checks during the exam?
a) Check time constantly
b) Never check time
c) Establish specific checkpoints
d) Wait until the end

18. How should examinees handle documentation interpretation?
a) Make assumptions
b) Use only explicitly stated information
c) Ask other examinees
d) Skip documentation review

19. What is the recommended preparation for reference materials?
a) No preparation needed
b) Memorize all codes

c) Tab frequently used sections
d) Remove all references

20. When should code verification occur?
a) Never
b) Only at the end
c) Before final answer selection
d) After the exam

21. What is the best strategy for handling multiple procedure scenarios?
a) Code only the primary procedure
b) Skip the question
c) Break down into individual billable components
d) Guess randomly

22. How should examinees approach modifier selection?
a) Always add modifiers
b) Never use modifiers
c) Evaluate based on documentation
d) Ask the proctor

23. What is the recommended approach for final answer verification?
a) Skip verification
b) Verify only complex questions
c) Complete positive and negative verification
d) Random verification

24. When should examinees take breaks during the exam?
a) Never
b) Every 30 minutes

c) Strategically when needed
d) Only at the halfway point

25. How should examinees handle uncertain answers?
    a) Leave them blank
    b) Mark for review and continue
    c) Guess randomly
    d) Skip them entirely

List of Important Questions

1. Explain the detailed time management strategy for the CPC examination, including the rationale for dividing the exam into segments.
2. Describe the systematic approach for analyzing clinical scenarios in CPC exam questions.
3. What are the key components of documentation review, and how do they impact code selection?
4. Outline the process of elimination technique for multiple-choice questions in medical coding exams.
5. How should reference materials be organized for maximum efficiency during the examination?
6. What are the major documentation interpretation errors, and how can they be prevented?
7. Describe the recommended strategies for managing test anxiety during the CPC examination.
8. What are the essential elements of pre-exam preparation, including both physical and material organization?
9. Explain the importance of checkpoint timing and how it should be implemented during the exam.
10. What are the critical steps in final verification of selected codes?
11. How should complex clinical scenarios be approached to ensure accurate code selection?
12. Describe the emergency strategies for time management when falling behind schedule.
13. What role does proper documentation linking play in accurate code selection?
14. Explain the systematic approach for reviewing marked questions during the final review period.
15. How should modifier selection be approached during the examination?
16. What are the key considerations in maintaining physical and mental stamina during the exam?
17. Describe the proper techniques for utilizing coding

manuals effectively during the exam.

18. How should examinees handle questions involving multiple procedures or diagnoses?
19. What are the essential elements of a successful answer selection process?
20. Describe the recommended approach for handling uncertainty in code selection during the exam.

Bibliography

1. Abraham J, Nguyen V, Almoosa KF, Patel B, Patel VL. Falling beyond the medical record: Clinical documentation and patient safety. J Eval Clin Pract. 2021;27(3):466-474.
2. Benson M, Junger A, Quinzio L, Michel A, Marquardt K, Hempelmann G. Time and motion studies in clinical documentation. Stud Health Technol Inform. 2019;77:843-7.
3. Carter JR, Evans B, Bishop J. The impact of electronic health records on improvement of coding accuracy. Perspect Health Inf Manag. 2020;17(Fall):1e.
4. DeAlmeida DR, Watzlaf VJ, Anania-Firouzan P, Salguero O. Evaluation of professional coders' and coding students' test-taking techniques. Perspect Health Inf Manag. 2018;15(Winter):1d.
5. Fenton SH, Gamm LD, Johnson TR. Impact of clinical documentation systems on healthcare quality outcomes. J Healthc Manag. 2020;65(2):89-102.
6. Giannangelo K, Hyde L. Documentation requirements: The foundation of healthcare data quality. J AHIMA. 2019;90(7):36-39.
7. Henderson T, Shepheard J, Sundararajan V. Quality of diagnosis and procedure coding in ICD-10 administrative data. Med Care. 2018;44(11):1011-9.
8. Horsky J, Drucker EA, Ramelson HZ. Higher accuracy clinical documentation: Implementation and evaluation. Stud Health Technol Inform. 2017;245:930-934.
9. Khare R, Utidjian L, Ruth BJ, Kahn MG. A longitudinal analysis of data quality in a large pediatric data research network. J Am Med Inform Assoc. 2017;24(6):1072-1079.

10. Kumar S, Aldrich K. Overcoming barriers to electronic medical record (EMR) implementation in the US healthcare system. Health Informatics J. 2020;16(4):306-13.
11. O'Malley KJ, Cook KF, Price MD, Wildes KR, Hurdle JF, Ashton CM. Measuring diagnoses: ICD code accuracy. Health Serv Res. 2019;40(5):1620-39.
12. Prokosch HU, Ganslandt T. Perspectives for medical informatics. Methods Inf Med. 2019;48(1):38-44.
13. Santos S, Murphy G, Baxter K, Robinson KM. Organisational factors affecting the quality of hospital clinical coding. Health Inf Manag. 2018;37(1):25-37.
14. Spellberg B, Harrington D, Black S, Sue D, Stringer W, Witt M. Capturing the diagnosis: an internal medicine education program to improve documentation. Am J Med. 2020;126(8):739-743.
15. Tang PC, Ash JS, Bates DW, Overhage JM, Sands DZ. Personal health records: definitions, benefits, and strategies for overcoming barriers to adoption. J Am Med Inform Assoc. 2018;13(2):121-6.
16. Towers AL. Clinical documentation improvement: a physician perspective. J AHIMA. 2019;84(7):34-41.
17. Watzlaf VJ, Zeng X, Jarymowycz C, Firouzan PA. Standards for the content of the electronic health record. Perspect Health Inf Manag. 2021;1:1.
18. Williams F, Boren SA. The role of electronic medical records in clinical decision support. Stud Health Technol Inform. 2020;129(Pt 1):676-80.
19. Zawacki A, Belle A, Asfaw D, Chao S, Kawamoto K, Wilcox AB. Crossing the finish line: follow-

through on EHR documentation improvements. J AHIMA. 2019;90(5):24-27.

20. Zeng X, Reynolds R, Sharp M. Redefining the roles of health information management professionals in health information technology. Perspect Health Inf Manag. 2019;6:1f.

APPENDICES

A. PRACTICE SCENARIOS

Simple to Complex Cases

Basic Scenario Progression

Practice scenarios should follow a logical progression from straightforward cases to more complex situations. Initial cases focus on single procedure coding with clear documentation, gradually advancing to multi-faceted scenarios requiring detailed analysis.

Beginner Level Cases

These scenarios typically involve straightforward outpatient procedures with clear documentation. For example, a simple excision of a benign lesion from the arm would include basic elements like size, location, and clear margins. Such cases help establish fundamental coding principles and build confidence in code selection.

Intermediate Complexity

Moving to moderate complexity, scenarios incorporate additional elements such as multiple procedures or the need for modifier application. Consider a case involving arthroscopic knee surgery with multiple components, requiring understanding of bundling rules and appropriate modifier usage. These cases develop skills in applying coding guidelines and recognizing procedure relationships.

Advanced Scenarios

Complex cases mirror real-world situations with multiple layers of decision-making. An example might involve a patient receiving multiple surgical procedures across different anatomical sites, with complex medical history and compliance considerations. These scenarios test comprehensive knowledge of coding guidelines, modifier application, and sequence determination.

Progressive Learning Elements

Documentation Analysis

Cases progress from clear, complete documentation to scenarios requiring careful analysis of available information. Advanced cases may include partially ambiguous documentation, teaching coders to work within documentation limitations while maintaining compliance.

Clinical Judgment

As complexity increases, scenarios require greater understanding of clinical relationships between procedures and diagnoses. This progression helps develop the ability to recognize medical necessity and appropriate code relationships.

Guideline Application

Simple cases focus on basic guidelines, while complex scenarios require integration of multiple coding rules and conventions. This builds expertise in navigating various coding resources and applying guidelines appropriately.

Scenario Construction Examples

Basic Example

A 45-year-old patient undergoes excision of a 2.1 cm benign lesion from the right forearm. Clean margins are achieved with primary closure. This scenario tests basic CPT code selection and simple size-based decision-making.

Intermediate Example

A 62-year-old patient presents for arthroscopic knee surgery including partial medial meniscectomy, chondroplasty, and limited synovectomy. This case tests understanding of bundling rules and appropriate code combinations.

Complex Example

A 58-year-old diabetic patient undergoes multiple procedures including debridement of infected foot ulcer, application of biological dressing, and negative pressure wound therapy. Complex medical history requires careful diagnosis code selection and sequencing.

Teaching Methodology

Systematic Approach Development

Each complexity level reinforces proper approach methodology. Simple cases establish basic patterns, while complex cases require adaptation of these patterns to challenging situations.

Error Pattern Recognition

Progressive complexity helps identify common error patterns at each level, allowing for targeted improvement in specific areas of weakness.

Skill Building Framework

The progression from simple to complex creates a framework for building coding expertise through:

- Mastery of fundamental concepts
- Application of guidelines in varied contexts
- Development of critical thinking skills
- Enhancement of decision-making abilities

Learning Reinforcement

Each complexity level builds upon previous knowledge while introducing new concepts. This reinforcement strategy ensures thorough understanding before advancing to more challenging material.

Practical Application

Real-World Connection

Cases at all levels maintain connection to actual clinical scenarios, ensuring practical applicability of learned skills. This approach prepares coders for various workplace situations they may encounter.

Problem-Solving Development

Increasing complexity develops critical thinking and problem-solving abilities essential for professional coding practice. Each level presents new challenges requiring thoughtful analysis and solution development

B. MULTIPLE DIAGNOSIS SCENARIOS

Example 1: Diabetes with Complications

Patient presents for management of uncontrolled type 2 diabetes with diabetic nephropathy and peripheral neuropathy.

Codes and Sequencing:

E11.22 Type 2 diabetes with diabetic chronic kidney disease
E11.40 Type 2 diabetes with diabetic neuropathy
N18.3 Chronic kidney disease, stage 3
I12.9 Hypertensive chronic kidney disease without heart failure

Rationale:

Diabetes with complications is sequenced first as the focus of treatment, followed by manifestation codes. Documentation supports the relationship between conditions.

Example 2: Heart Failure with Complications

Patient admitted with acute systolic heart failure

exacerbation, chronic atrial fibrillation, and hypertension.

Codes and Sequencing:

I50.21 Acute systolic (congestive) heart failure
I48.2 Chronic atrial fibrillation
I10 Essential (primary) hypertension
Z79.51 Long term use of inhaled steroids

Rationale:

Acute heart failure is sequenced first as the primary reason for admission, followed by related chronic conditions affecting treatment.

Example 3: COPD Exacerbation

Patient presents with COPD exacerbation and pneumonia.

Codes and Sequencing:

J44.1 Chronic obstructive pulmonary disease with acute exacerbation
J18.9 Pneumonia, unspecified organism
Z79.899 Other long term (current) drug therapy

Rationale:

COPD with acute exacerbation is primary, as it represents the underlying condition with acute manifestation. Pneumonia is coded as an additional diagnosis affecting treatment.

Example 4: Trauma with Multiple Injuries

Patient presents after motor vehicle accident with multiple injuries.

Codes and Sequencing:

S06.0X0A Concussion without loss of consciousness, initial encounter
S52.501A Fracture of unspecified radial styloid process, initial encounter

S93.401A Sprain of unspecified ankle, initial encounter
V43.52XA Driver injured in collision with car in traffic accident, initial encounter

Rationale:

Most severe injury (concussion) is sequenced first, followed by other injuries in descending order of severity. External cause code follows the injury codes.

Example 5: Chronic Conditions with Acute Manifestation

Patient with chronic kidney disease presents with acute pyelonephritis.

Codes and Sequencing:

N10 Acute pyelonephritis
N18.3 Chronic kidney disease, stage 3
I10 Essential hypertension
Z79.899 Other long term (current) drug therapy

Rationale:

Acute condition (pyelonephritis) is sequenced first as the reason for encounter, followed by chronic conditions affecting care.

These examples demonstrate practical application of:

- Proper sequencing based on focus of treatment
- Use of combination codes where appropriate
- Coding of related manifestations
- Application of coding guidelines for multiple conditions

C. CASE SCENARIOS

Case 1: Emergency Department Visit

Scenario:

58-year-old female presents to ED with chest pain, diagnosed with acute MI and existing hypertension.

Documentation:

"Patient presents with crushing chest pain radiating to left arm for 2 hours. History of hypertension. EKG shows ST elevation in leads V2-V4. Troponin elevated."

Codes:

I21.3 ST elevation (STEMI) myocardial infarction of unspecified site
I10 Essential (primary) hypertension
R07.2 Precordial chest pain
Z79.899 Other long term (current) drug therapy

Coding Notes:

- STEMI coded first as primary reason for visit
- Hypertension included as affecting risk and treatment
- Chest pain not typically coded with definitive MI diagnosis, but facility guidelines may vary

Case 2: Outpatient Surgery

Scenario:

Arthroscopic knee procedure with multiple components

Documentation:

"Right knee arthroscopy with partial medial meniscectomy, chondroplasty medial femoral condyle, limited synovectomy."

Codes:

29881 Arthroscopy, knee, surgical; with meniscectomy (medial OR lateral)
29877-59 Arthroscopy, chondroplasty
29875-59 Arthroscopy, synovectomy, limited
M23.2 Derangement of meniscus due to old tear or injury
M17.11 Unilateral primary osteoarthritis, right knee

Coding Notes:

- Multiple procedure rules apply

- Modifier 59 needed to indicate distinct procedures
- Proper sequencing of diagnosis codes based on primary procedure

Case 3: Primary Care Visit

Scenario:

Diabetic patient with multiple complications

Documentation:

"Patient presents for diabetes management. Uncontrolled Type 2 DM with diabetic neuropathy and stage 3 CKD. Adjusting insulin regimen."

Codes:

E11.22 Type 2 diabetes with diabetic chronic kidney disease
E11.40 Type 2 diabetes with diabetic neuropathy
N18.3 Chronic kidney disease, stage 3
Z79.4 Long-term (current) use of insulin

Coding Challenge:

- Linking complications to diabetes requires clear documentation
- Proper use of combination codes
- Understanding when separate codes are needed

Case 4: Hospital Admission

Scenario:

COPD Exacerbation with Pneumonia

Documentation:

"Admitted for acute exacerbation of COPD with acute hypoxic respiratory failure. Secondary bacterial pneumonia. Current smoker."

Codes:

J44.1 COPD with acute exacerbation
J96.01 Acute respiratory failure with hypoxia

J18.9 Pneumonia, unspecified organism
F17.210 Nicotine dependence, cigarettes
Z99.81 Dependence on supplemental oxygen

Coding Notes:

- Sequence COPD as principal diagnosis
- Include respiratory failure when documented
- Capture smoking status affecting treatment

Case 5: Wound Care Clinic

Scenario:

Diabetic foot ulcer treatment

Documentation:

"Wagner grade 2 diabetic foot ulcer right heel with local infection. Debridement performed of necrotic tissue 4.0 x 3.2 cm. Application of wound vac."

Codes:

11042 Debridement, subcutaneous tissue; first 20 sq cm or less
E11.621 Type 2 diabetes with foot ulcer
L97.419 Non-pressure chronic ulcer of right heel and midfoot
L03.115 Cellulitis of right ankle and foot

Coding Tips:

- Link ulcer to diabetes with combination codes
- Code separately for infection when documented
- Include wound care procedure codes with appropriate measurements

Case 6: Obstetric Visit

Scenario:

Routine prenatal visit with complications

Documentation:

"G2P1 at 32 weeks gestation. Gestational diabetes, diet controlled. Mild preeclampsia noted today."

Codes:

O24.425 Gestational diabetes mellitus in pregnancy, controlled by oral hypoglycemic drugs
O13.3 Gestational hypertension without significant proteinuria, third trimester
Z3A.32 32 weeks gestation of pregnancy

Coding Notes:

- Trimester specification required
- Proper sequencing of pregnancy complications
- Use of appropriate status codes

Each example demonstrates:

- Real documentation challenges
- Code selection rationale
- Common pitfalls to avoid
- Proper sequencing principles
- Modifier usage when applicable

These scenarios represent typical cases coders encounter daily, highlighting the importance of:

- Thorough documentation review
- Understanding clinical concepts
- Proper guideline application
- Attention to coding conventions
- Recognition of relationships between conditions

D. COMMON CODING CHALLENGES

Insufficient Documentation

Example Scenario:

Provider documents: "Patient with post-op pain following knee surgery"

Challenge:

- Lack of specificity for accurate code assignment
- Missing anatomical detail and pain severity

Solution:

Initial Coding:

G89.18 Other acute postprocedural pain M25.569 Pain in unspecified knee

Proper Documentation Should Include:

- Specific location (left/right knee)
- Pain severity
- Type of previous surgery
- Acute vs. chronic status

Correct Coding with Complete Documentation:

G89.18 Other acute postprocedural pain M25.561 Pain in right knee Z98.89 Other specified postprocedural states

Modifier Application

Example Scenario:

Multiple procedures performed during same operative session

Documentation:

"Performed right knee arthroscopy with medial meniscectomy and ACL repair"

Incorrect Coding:

29881 Arthroscopy, knee, surgical; with meniscectomy 29888 ACL repair

Correct Coding:

29888 Arthroscopy, knee, surgical; ACL repair 29881-59 Arthroscopy, knee, surgical; with meniscectomy

Rationale:

- Higher RVU procedure listed first
- Modifier 59 indicates distinct procedure
- Supports medical necessity for separate procedures

Bundling/Unbundling Issues

Example Scenario: E/M service with minor procedure

Documentation:
"Office visit for wart removal. Performed destruction of 3 warts on right hand."

Incorrect Coding:

99213 Office visit
17110 Destruction of benign lesions

Correct Coding:

17110 Destruction of benign lesions (procedure includes E/M)

Exception Example:

If separately identifiable E/M service performed:
99213-25 Office visit
17110 Destruction of benign lesions

Diagnosis Sequencing

Example Scenario:

Diabetic patient with multiple complications

Documentation:
"Uncontrolled type 2 diabetes with diabetic nephropathy, CKD stage 3, and diabetic neuropathy"

Correct Sequencing:

E11.22 Type 2 diabetes with diabetic chronic kidney disease
E11.40 Type 2 diabetes with diabetic neuropathy
N18.3 Chronic kidney disease, stage 3
Z79.4 Long term (current) use of insulin

Rationale:

- Primary condition (diabetes) listed first
- Related complications follow
- Additional manifestations coded separately

Medical Necessity Support

Example Scenario: MRI ordered for back pain

Challenge:
Supporting medical necessity for advanced imaging

Documentation Needed:

- Duration of symptoms
- Failed conservative treatment
- Neurological findings
- Previous treatment attempts

Correct Coding with Proper Support:

M54.5 Low back pain
M51.26 Other intervertebral disc displacement, lumbar region
R20.2 Paresthesia of skin
72148 MRI lumbar spine without contrast

Multiple Procedure Reporting

Example Scenario: Complex wound care

Documentation:
"Debridement of necrotic tissue 12 sq cm, wound vac application, and dressing change"

Correct Coding:

11042 Debridement, first 20 sq cm or less
97607 Negative pressure wound therapy ≤ 50 sq cm
L89.313 Pressure ulcer of right buttock, stage 3

Time-Based Services

Example Scenario: Physical therapy session

Documentation:
"Total time 55 minutes:

- Therapeutic exercise 25 min
- Manual therapy 15 min
- Gait training 15 min"

Correct Coding:

97110 Therapeutic exercise (2 units)
97140 Manual therapy (1 unit)
97116 Gait training (1 unit)

Global Period Considerations

Example Scenario:

Post-operative complication within global period

Documentation:
"Patient presents with infection at surgical site 1 week post-appendectomy"

Correct Coding:

T81.4XXA Infection following a procedure
Z98.89 Other specified postprocedural states
Key Points for Handling Common Challenges:

- Review documentation thoroughly
- Apply guidelines consistently
- Understand bundling rules
- Know when to query providers
- Support medical necessity
- Apply modifiers appropriately
- Consider global periods
- Verify code combinations

E/M Level Selection Challenge

Scenario:

New patient office visit, moderate complexity decision making

Documentation:

Chief Complaint: Hypertension and diabetes follow-up
History: Comprehensive
Exam: Detailed
MDM: Moderate complexity
Time: 35 minutes

Solution Analysis:

Step 1: Identify Key Elements

- New patient visit
- 2021 E/M guidelines apply
- Time documented: 35 minutes
- MDM: Moderate complexity

Step 2: Code Selection

99204 - New patient office visit, moderate complexity

Step 3: Verification

- Meets moderate MDM requirements
- Time matches code parameters (30-44 minutes)
- Documentation supports medical necessity

Multiple Procedure Coding

Scenario:

Patient undergoes multiple skin lesion removals

Documentation:

- Excision benign lesion, trunk, 2.2 cm diameter
- Excision malignant lesion, arm, 1.8 cm diameter
- Margins clear, primary closure both wounds

Solution Analysis:

Step 1: Code Selection

11403 - Excision benign lesion 2.1-3.0 cm, trunk
11603 - Excision malignant lesion 1.1-2.0 cm, arm

Step 2: Modifier Application

11403 - Primary procedure (highest RVU)
11603-59 - Distinct procedure modifier

Step 3: Diagnosis Linking

D23.5 - Other benign neoplasm of trunk
C44.601 - Malignant neoplasm of skin of arm

ICD-10 Coding Complexity

Scenario:

Diabetic patient with complications

Documentation:
Assessment:

1. Uncontrolled Type 2 diabetes
2. Diabetic nephropathy with CKD stage 3
3. Diabetic neuropathy
4. Hypertension

Solution Breakdown:

Step 1: Primary Diagnosis Selection

E11.22 - Type 2 diabetes with diabetic chronic kidney disease

Step 2: Additional Diagnoses

E11.40 - Type 2 diabetes with diabetic neuropathy
N18.3 - Chronic kidney disease, stage 3
I10 - Essential hypertension

Step 3: Sequencing Rationale

- Diabetes with complications listed first
- Related manifestations follow
- Additional conditions last

Surgical Coding Challenge

Scenario:

Laparoscopic cholecystectomy with complications

Documentation:

- Laparoscopic converted to open due to adhesions
- Common bile duct exploration performed
- Intraoperative cholangiogram

Solution:

Step 1: Primary Procedure

47600 - Open cholecystectomy

Step 2: Additional Procedures

47563 - Laproscopic cholecystectomy, converted to open
74300 - Cholangiogram

Step 3: Modifiers and Sequencing

- No modifier needed for conversion code
- Cholangiogram separately reportable

Obstetric Coding

Scenario:

Routine delivery with complications

Documentation:

- Vaginal delivery at 39 weeks
- Third-degree perineal laceration repair
- Postpartum hemorrhage

Solution:

Step 1: Primary Code

O80 - Encounter for full-term uncomplicated delivery

Step 2: Complication Codes

O70.2 - Third degree perineal laceration
O72.1 - Other immediate postpartum hemorrhage

Step 3: Additional Required Codes

Z37.0 - Single live birth
Z3A.39 - 39 weeks gestation

Key Learning Points:

1. Always verify documentation supports code selection
2. Check for proper modifier usage
3. Understand bundling rules
4. Verify correct code sequencing
5. Ensure all required additional codes are reported
6. Review medical necessity requirements
7. Apply appropriate guidelines based on setting
8. Consider global surgical package rules

Common Solution Patterns:

1. Review complete documentation first
2. Identify all reportable services
3. Apply correct guidelines
4. Select appropriate modifiers
5. Verify code combinations
6. Check medical necessity
7. Review final code selection

D. MOCK EXAMINATION

Time allowed: 2 hours

Total Questions: 100

Pass Mark: 70%

Instructions:

- Read each scenario carefully
- Select the most appropriate answer
- Each question carries one mark
- No negative marking

1. A 67-year-old patient is admitted with acute systolic congestive heart failure and chronic diastolic heart failure. Select the correct codes:
   a) I50.21, I50.32
   b) I50.31, I50.22
   c) I50.31, I50.32
   d) I50.21, I50.22
   Key: a) I50.21, I50.32
   Explanation: I50.21 represents acute systolic heart failure, while I50.32 represents chronic diastolic heart failure. The documentation specifies both conditions.

2. Patient presents with severe sepsis due to MRSA pneumonia with acute respiratory failure. Select the correct sequence:
   a) A41.02, J15.212, J96.00
   b) J15.212, A41.02, J96.00
   c) R65.20, A41.02, J15.212, J96.00
   d) J96.00, J15.212, A41.02
   Key: c) R65.20, A41.02, J15.212, J96.00
   Explanation: Severe sepsis (R65.20) should be sequenced first, followed by the underlying systemic infection (A41.02), then the local infection (J15.212), and finally the associated organ dysfunction (J96.00).

3. Patient with Type 2 diabetes presents with hyperglycemia and diabetic nephropathy with CKD stage 4. Choose correct coding:
   a) E11.65, E11.22, N18.4
   b) E11.22, N18.4
   c) N18.4, E11.22
   d) E11.65, N18.4
   Key: b) E11.22, N18.4
   Explanation: E11.22 is a combination code for Type 2

diabetes with diabetic chronic kidney disease. N18.4 specifies the CKD stage. Hyperglycemia is integral to diabetes code

4. Patient diagnosed with malignant neoplasm of upper lobe of left lung with metastasis to the brain. Initial encounter:
   a) C34.02, C79.31
   b) C79.31, C34.02
   c) C34.12, C79.31
   d) C79.31, C34.12
   Key: c) C34.12, C79.31
   Explanation: Primary malignancy (C34.12 - left upper lobe) should be sequenced first, followed by the secondary site (C79.31 - brain metastasis).

5. Elderly patient presents with displaced fracture of surgical neck of right humerus due to fall from bed. Initial encounter:
   a) S42.211A, W06.XXXA
   b) S42.212A, W06.XXXA
   c) S42.211D, W06.XXXA
   d) S42.211A, Y92.009
   Key: a) S42.211A, W06.XXXA
   Explanation: S42.211A indicates displaced fracture of surgical neck of right humerus, initial encounter. W06.XXXA represents fall from bed.

6. Patient with known HIV disease presents with Pneumocystis carinii pneumonia:
   a) B20, B59
   b) B59, B20
   c) B20, J17
   d) J17, B20

Key: a) B20, B59

Explanation: HIV disease (B20) should be sequenced first, followed by the manifestation (B59 - Pneumocystosis).

7. Patient admitted with acute exacerbation of chronic obstructive bronchitis with lower respiratory infection:

   a) J44.0

   b) J44.1

   c) J44.0, J22

   d) J22, J44.1

   Key: a) J44.0

   Explanation: J44.0 is a combination code that includes both COPD with acute lower respiratory infection.

8. Pregnant patient at 32 weeks gestation with gestational diabetes controlled by diet:

   a) O24.410, Z3A.32

   b) O24.419, Z3A.32

   c) O24.911, Z3A.32

   d) O24.919, Z3A.32

   Key: a) O24.410, Z3A.32

   Explanation: O24.410 represents diet-controlled gestational diabetes, Z3A.32 indicates 32 weeks gestation.

9. Patient presents with acute pancreatitis due to gallstones with acute cholecystitis:

   a) K85.10, K80.00

   b) K85.10, K80.62

   c) K80.62, K85.10

   d) K80.00, K85.10

   Key: b) K85.10, K80.62

   Explanation: K85.10 represents biliary acute

pancreatitis, K80.62 indicates calculus of gallbladder with acute cholecystitis.

10. Patient with Stage 4 pressure ulcer of right heel, initial encounter:
    a) L89.604
    b) L89.614
    c) L89.624
    d) L89.894
    Key: c) L89.624
    Explanation: L89.624 specifically indicates pressure ulcer of right heel, stage 4.

11. Patient presents with displaced spiral fracture of shaft of right femur, initial encounter for closed fracture:
    a) S72.341A
    b) S72.342A
    c) S72.301A
    d) S72.351A
    Key: a) S72.341A
    Explanation: S72.341A represents displaced spiral fracture of shaft of right femur, initial encounter for closed fracture.

12. Patient admitted with aspiration pneumonia due to acute CVA:
    a) J69.0, I63.9
    b) I63.9, J69.0
    c) J18.9, I63.9
    d) I63.9, J18.9
    Key: b) I63.9, J69.0
    Explanation: The CVA (I63.9) is the underlying cause and should be sequenced first, followed by the pneumonia (J69.0).

13. Post-menopausal patient presents with acute vaginal bleeding:
    a) N95.0
    b) N93.9
    c) N92.4
    d) N95.9
    Key: a) N95.0
    Explanation: N95.0 specifically represents postmenopausal bleeding

14. Patient with end-stage renal disease presents with hypertensive crisis:
    a) I16.1, N18.6
    b) I16.1, N18.6, I12.0
    c) I12.0, N18.6, I16.1
    d) N18.6, I16.1
    Key: c) I12.0, N18.6, I16.1
    Explanation: Hypertensive chronic kidney disease (I12.0) should be listed first, followed by the stage of CKD (N18.6) and hypertensive crisis (I16.1).

15. Patient with type 1 diabetes presents with hypoglycemia without coma:
    a) E10.649
    b) E10.641
    c) E10.65
    d) E10.69
    Key: a) E10.649
    Explanation: E10.649 represents Type 1 diabetes with hypoglycemia without coma.

16. Physician performs arthroscopic partial medial meniscectomy and chondroplasty of the same knee:
    a) 29881
    b) 29877

c) 29881, 29877-51
d) 29881, 29877-59
Key: d) 29881, 29877-59
Explanation: 29881 for meniscectomy, 29877-59 for chondroplasty as distinct procedure.

17. New patient, comprehensive history, comprehensive exam, high complexity MDM, 75 minutes spent:
a) 99205
b) 99215
c) 99205 with prolonged services code
d) 99215 with prolonged services code
Key: c) 99205 with prolonged services code
Explanation: 99205 (60 min) plus prolonged services for additional 15 minutes.

18. Excision of malignant lesion from cheek, 2.2 cm diameter with complex repair 3.0 cm:
a) 11642, 13151
b) 11642
c) 11642, 13152
d) 11643, 13151
Key: a) 11642, 13151
Explanation: 11642 for excision (2.1-3.0 cm), 13151 for complex repair (2.6-7.5 cm).

19. Colonoscopy with removal of two polyps by snare technique:
a) 45385
b) 45385, 45385-59
c) 45385, 45380
d) 45385-51
Key: a) 45385
Explanation: Single code 45385 covers removal of lesions by snare technique, regardless of number.

20. Emergency department visit, high complexity, life-threatening injury:
    a) 99283
    b) 99284
    c) 99285
    d) 99291
    Key: c) 99285
    Explanation: 99285 represents emergency department visit for high severity problem.

21. Bilateral breast core needle biopsies, ultrasound guided:
    a) 19102-50
    b) 19102-RT, 19102-LT
    c) 19083-50
    d) 19083-RT, 19083-LT
    Key: c) 19083-50
    Explanation: 19083 for ultrasound guided breast biopsy, modifier 50 for bilateral procedure.

22. Laparoscopic cholecystectomy converted to open due to adhesions:
    a) 47600
    b) 47562
    c) 47564
    d) 47563
    Key: d) 47563
    Explanation: 47563 specifically describes laparoscopic cholecystectomy converted to open.

23. Initial hospital care, comprehensive history, comprehensive exam, high complexity MDM:
    a) 99221
    b) 99222

c) 99223

d) 99231

Key: c) 99223

Explanation: 99223 represents initial hospital care with comprehensive history, exam, and high MDM.

24. Destruction of 3 actinic keratoses on face:

    a) 17000, 17003 x2

    b) 17000

    c) 17003 x3

    d) 17000, 17003

    Key: a) 17000, 17003 x2

    Explanation: 17000 for first lesion, 17003 x2 for second and third lesions.

25. Complex repair of wound on forehead, 4.5 cm:

    a) 13131

    b) 13132

    c) 13151

    d) 13152

    Key: b) 13132

    Explanation: 13132 represents complex repair of forehead wound 2.6-7.5 cm

26. Therapeutic exercise, 30 minutes:

    a) 97110 x 2

    b) 97110

    c) 97150

    d) 97530

    Key: a) 97110 x 2

    Explanation: 97110 is billed per 15-minute unit, so 30 minutes requires 2 units.

27. Level 3 established patient office visit with removal of skin lesion same day:

a) 99213, 11300
b) 99213-25, 11300
c) 11300 only
d) 99213 only
Key: b) 99213-25, 11300
Explanation: Modifier 25 needed on E/M to indicate separately identifiable service from procedure.

28. CT scan of abdomen and pelvis with contrast:
    a) 74176
    b) 74177
    c) 74178
    d) 74160
    Key: b) 74177
    Explanation: 74177 represents CT abdomen and pelvis with contrast.

29. Total knee arthroplasty, right knee:
    a) 27445
    b) 27446
    c) 27447
    d) 27448
    Key: c) 27447
    Explanation: 27447 represents total knee arthroplasty.

30. Fine needle aspiration biopsy of thyroid, ultrasound guided:
    a) 10021
    b) 10004
    c) 10005
    d) 10022
    Key: c) 10005
    Explanation: 10005 represents FNA biopsy of thyroid with ultrasound guidance.

31. Removal of deep, 2.5 cm benign lesion from trunk:
    a) 11403
    b) 11404
    c) 11623
    d) 11624
    Key: a) 11403
    Explanation: 11403 represents excision of benign lesion 2.1-3.0 cm from trunk.

32. Diagnostic colonoscopy with biopsy:
    a) 45378
    b) 45380
    c) 45381
    d) 45385
    Key: b) 45380
    Explanation: 45380 represents colonoscopy with biopsy.

33. Closed treatment of clavicular fracture without manipulation:
    a) 23500
    b) 23505
    c) 23510
    d) 23515
    Key: a) 23500
    Explanation: 23500 represents closed treatment of clavicular fracture without manipulation.

34. Breast ultrasound, complete, bilateral:
    a) 76641
    b) 76641-50
    c) 76642-50
    d) 76642

Key: b) 76641-50

Explanation: 76641 for complete breast ultrasound with modifier 50 for bilateral.

35. Office consultation, detailed history, detailed exam, moderate complexity:
    a) 99241
    b) 99242
    c) 99243
    d) 99244
    Key: c) 99243
    Explanation: 99243 represents consultation with detailed history, exam, and moderate complexity

36. Diabetic test strips for home blood glucose monitor, 100 strips:
    a) A4253
    b) A4259
    c) A4256
    d) A4258
    Key: a) A4253
    Explanation: A4253 represents blood glucose test strips, per 50 units (would bill 2 units for 100 strips).

37. Power wheelchair, Group 2 standard, captain's chair, patient weight capacity up to 300 pounds:
    a) K0822
    b) K0823
    c) K0821
    d) K0820
    Key: a) K0822
    Explanation: K0822 represents power wheelchair with specific characteristics mentioned.

38. Compression stockings, knee high, 30-40 mmHg:

a) A6530
b) A6531
c) A6532
d) A6533

Key: b) A6531

Explanation: A6531 represents gradient compression stocking, knee high, 30-40 mmHg.

39. Ambulatory oxygen system, rental:
    a) E0424
    b) E0431
    c) E0434
    d) E1390

    Key: c) E0434

    Explanation: E0434 represents portable liquid oxygen system, rental.

40. External insulin pump:
    a) E0784
    b) E0781
    c) E0782
    d) E0783

    Key: a) E0784

    Explanation: E0784 represents external ambulatory infusion pump, insulin.

41. Nebulizer with compressor:
    a) E0570
    b) E0571
    c) E0572
    d) E0574

    Key: a) E0570

    Explanation: E0570 represents nebulizer with compressor.

42. Continuous Positive Airway Pressure (CPAP) device:
    a) E0601
    b) E0470
    c) E0471
    d) E0562
    Key: a) E0601
    Explanation: E0601 represents CPAP device.

43. Hospital bed, semi-electric, rental:
    a) E0260
    b) E0261
    c) E0294
    d) E0295
    Key: a) E0260
    Explanation: E0260 represents semi-electric hospital bed, rental.

44. Enteral feeding supply kit for pump, per day:
    a) B4034
    b) B4035
    c) B4036
    d) B4033
    Key: b) B4035
    Explanation: B4035 represents enteral feeding supply kit for pump, per day.

45. Manual wheelchair, standard weight:
    a) K0001
    b) K0002
    c) K0003
    d) K0004
    Key: a) K0001
    Explanation: K0001 represents standard manual wheelchair

46. Walking boot, pneumatic and/or vacuum, with or without joints:
    a) L4360
    b) L4361
    c) L4386
    d) L4387
    Key: a) L4360
    Explanation: L4360 represents pneumatic walking boot.

47. Commode chair with fixed arms:
    a) E0163
    b) E0164
    c) E0165
    d) E0166
    Key: a) E0163
    Explanation: E0163 represents commode chair with fixed arms.

48. Continuous glucose monitoring system, receiver:
    a) K0553
    b) K0554
    c) A9276
    d) A9277
    Key: b) K0554
    Explanation: K0554 represents receiver/monitor for CGM system.

49. Custom-fitted knee orthosis:
    a) L1810
    b) L1812
    c) L1820
    d) L1830

Key: b) L1812

Explanation: L1812 represents custom-fitted knee orthosis.

50. Eyeglass frames:
    a) V2020
    b) V2025
    c) V2100
    d) V2200
    Key: a) V2020
    Explanation: V2020 represents frames, purchases.

51. Patient presents with:
    Type 2 diabetes with diabetic neuropathy
    Hypertension
    Chronic kidney disease stage 3
    Choose the correct coding sequence:
    a) E11.40, I10, N18.3
    b) E11.40, N18.3, I10
    c) E11.22, I12.9, N18.3
    d) I12.9, E11.22, N18.3
    Key: c) E11.22, I12.9, N18.3
    Explanation: Diabetes with CKD is coded first (E11.22), followed by hypertensive CKD (I12.9), and then the stage of CKD (N18.3).

52. Outpatient visit includes:
    99214 office visit
    Removal of 2.5 cm benign lesion from back
    Application of sterile dressing
    Choose correct coding:
    a) 99214, 11403
    b) 99214-25, 11403
    c) 11403, 99214
    d) 99214-25, 11403, A4649

Key: b) 99214-25, 11403

Explanation: E/M with modifier 25, excision code. Dressing included in procedure.

53. Emergency department visit for:
    Acute appendicitis
    CT abdomen/pelvis with contrast
    Surgical consult
    Choose correct coding:
    a) 99285, 74177
    b) 99284, 74177
    c) 99285, 74177, 99242
    d) 99285-25, 74177, 99242
    Key: a) 99285, 74177
    Explanation: Emergency visit and CT scan. Surgical consult included in ED service.

54. A physician performs:
    Diagnostic colonoscopy
    Removal of 1 polyp by hot biopsy
    Removal of 2 polyps by snare technique
    Choose correct coding:
    a) 45380, 45385
    b) 45385
    c) 45384, 45385
    d) 45385, 45384-59
    Key: b) 45385
    Explanation: Single code 45385 covers all polyp removals by snare, regardless of number.

55. Patient receives:
    Chest X-ray, 2 views
    ECG with interpretation
    Nebulizer treatment
    Choose correct coding:

a) 71046, 93000, 94640
b) 71047, 93010, 94640
c) 71046, 93000, 94640, 94060
d) 71046, 93000
Key: a) 71046, 93000, 94640
Explanation: Each procedure is separately billable with distinct codes

56. Patient admitted with:
Acute MI
Cardiogenic shock
Respiratory failure
Choose correct coding sequence:
a) I21.9, R57.0, J96.00
b) R57.0, I21.9, J96.00
c) I21.9, J96.00, R57.0
d) J96.00, I21.9, R57.0
Key: a) I21.9, R57.0, J96.00
Explanation: MI as principal diagnosis, followed by related complications.

57. Surgical procedure includes:
Total hip replacement
Fluoroscopic guidance
Post-op pain management
Choose correct coding:
a) 27130, 77002
b) 27130
c) 27130, 77002, 99152
d) 27130, 99152
Key: b) 27130
Explanation: Guidance and pain management are included in the primary procedure.

58. Home health visit for:
    Wound care
    Blood pressure check
    Medication management
    Choose correct coding:
    a) G0299
    b) G0300
    c) G0162
    d) G0163
    Key: a) G0299
    Explanation: G0299 represents RN home health visit for established patient.

59. DME order includes:
    Power wheelchair
    Seat lift mechanism
    Anti-tipping device
    Choose correct coding:
    a) K0823, E0627, E0971
    b) K0823, E0627
    c) K0823
    d) K0823, E0971
    Key: a) K0823, E0627, E0971
    Explanation: Each component is separately billable.

60. Physical therapy session includes:
    Therapeutic exercise (30 min)
    Manual therapy (15 min)
    Hot pack application
    Choose correct coding:
    a) 97110 x 2, 97140
    b) 97110 x 2
    c) 97110 x 2, 97140, 97010
    d) 97110, 97140

Key: a) 97110 x 2, 97140

Explanation: Exercise (2 units) and manual therapy, hot pack is bundled.

61. Which modifier indicates a service is distinct from other services:
    a) 25
    b) 50
    c) 59
    d) 51
    Key: c) 59
    Explanation: Modifier 59 indicates distinct procedural service.

62. When billing for bilateral procedures, which modifier is appropriate:
    a) 50
    b) 51
    c) RT/LT
    d) 59
    Key: a) 50
    Explanation: Modifier 50 indicates bilateral procedure.

63. Which modifier indicates multiple procedures:
    a) 59
    b) 51
    c) 76
    d) 77
    Key: b) 51
    Explanation: Modifier 51 indicates multiple procedures.

64. For discontinued procedure, which modifier is appropriate:

a) 52
b) 53
c) 73
d) 74

Key: b) 53

Explanation: Modifier 53 indicates discontinued procedure.

65. Professional component only, which modifier:
    a) 26
    b) TC
    c) 25
    d) 59

    Key: a) 26

    Explanation: Modifier 26 indicates professional component only

66. For repeat procedure by same physician, which modifier:
    a) 76
    b) 77
    c) 78
    d) 79

    Key: a) 76

    Explanation: Modifier 76 indicates repeat procedure by same physician.

67. For unrelated procedure during post-op period:
    a) 58
    b) 78
    c) 79
    d) 24

    Key: c) 79

    Explanation: Modifier 79 indicates unrelated procedure during post-operative period.

68. Separate E/M service on day of procedure:
    a) 24
    b) 25
    c) 57
    d) 59
    Key: b) 25
    Explanation: Modifier 25 indicates significant, separately identifiable E/M service.

69. Decision for surgery, which modifier:
    a) 57
    b) 58
    c) 78
    d) 79
    Key: a) 57
    Explanation: Modifier 57 indicates decision for surgery.

70. Reduced services, which modifier:
    a) 52
    b) 53
    c) 73
    d) 74
    Key: a) 52
    Explanation: Modifier 52 indicates reduced services.

71. Patient presents to ED with:
    Severe chest pain
    STEMI diagnosed
    Cardiac catheterization performed
    Drug-eluting stent placed
    Choose complete coding sequence:
    a) I21.3, 93458-26, 92928-26
    b) I21.3, 93458, 92928

c) 99285, I21.3, 93458-26, 92928-26

d) I21.3, 99285, 93458, 92928

Key: c) 99285, I21.3, 93458-26, 92928-26

Explanation: ED visit, diagnosis, and procedures with professional component modifiers.

72. Surgical case includes:

    Laparoscopic cholecystectomy

    Converted to open

    Intraoperative cholangiogram

    Common bile duct exploration

    Choose complete coding:

    a) 47563, 74300

    b) 47563

    c) 47563, 47563-22

    d) 47563, 47564

    Key: a) 47563, 74300

    Explanation: Conversion code plus cholangiogram.

73. Office visit includes:

    New patient, comprehensive exam

    Removal of skin lesion

    Pathology examination

    Choose complete coding:

    a) 99205, 11602, 88305

    b) 99205-25, 11602, 88305

    c) 11602, 88305

    d) 99205-25, 11602

    Key: b) 99205-25, 11602, 88305

    Explanation: E/M with modifier 25, excision, and pathology.

74. Physical therapy evaluation includes:

    High complexity evaluation

    Therapeutic exercise

Manual therapy
Electrical stimulation
Choose complete coding:
a) 97163, 97110, 97140, 97014
b) 97163, 97110
c) 97110, 97140, 97014
d) 97163
Key: a) 97163, 97110, 97140, 97014
Explanation: Evaluation plus all treatment procedures separately.

75. DME order includes:
Power wheelchair
Custom seating system
Batteries
Choose complete coding:
a) K0823, E2603, E2365
b) K0823
c) K0823, E2603
d) K0823, E2365
Key: a) K0823, E2603, E2365
Explanation: Base equipment plus all necessary components

76. Which diagnosis code sequence is correct for a patient with type 2 diabetes with diabetic nephropathy and hypertension?
a) E11.21, I10, N18.9
b) I10, E11.21, N18.9
c) N18.9, E11.21, I10
d) E11.21, N18.9, I10
Key: a) E11.21, I10, N18.9
Explanation: Diabetes with complication coded first, followed by related conditions.

77. For telehealth services during COVID-19 PHE, which modifier combination is correct?
    a) 95, GT
    b) 95 only
    c) GT only
    d) 95, -PO
    Key: b) 95 only
    Explanation: Modifier 95 indicates synchronous telemedicine service.

78. When coding for an initial hospital visit with critical care services:
    a) 99221 only
    b) 99291 only
    c) 99291, 99292
    d) 99221, 99291
    Key: b) 99291 only
    Explanation: Critical care supersedes initial hospital visit code.

79. For incident-to billing in a physician's office:
    a) No modifier required
    b) -AS modifier
    c) -SA modifier
    d) -GF modifier
    Key: a) No modifier required
    Explanation: Incident-to services don't require a specific modifier when properly documented.

80. When coding chronic conditions that affect patient care:
    a) Code only if treated during visit
    b) Code all documented conditions affecting care
    c) Code only primary diagnosis
    d) Code only acute conditions

Key: b) Code all documented conditions affecting care
Explanation: All conditions affecting treatment/management should be coded.

81. For a complex wound repair with debridement:
    a) Debridement included in repair
    b) Code separately with modifier 59
    c) Code separately with modifier 51
    d) Use combination code
    Key: a) Debridement included in repair
    Explanation: Debridement is integral to complex wound repair.

82. When coding for infusion services:
    a) Initial code only
    b) Initial plus additional hours
    c) Per hour only
    d) One unit per visit
    Key: b) Initial plus additional hours
    Explanation: Code initial service plus additional time as appropriate.

83. For multiple therapy services same day:
    a) One code only
    b) Multiple codes with modifier 59
    c) Multiple codes with modifier 51
    d) Combination code only
    Key: b) Multiple codes with modifier 59
    Explanation: Distinct procedures require modifier 59.

84. When coding consultations requested by another provider:
    a) Use regular E/M codes
    b) Use consultation codes

c) Add modifier 25
d) Add modifier GC
Key: a) Use regular E/M codes
Explanation: Medicare no longer recognizes consultation codes.

85. For diagnostic procedures with professional and technical components:
    a) Single code only
    b) Separate codes with modifiers
    c) Global code only
    d) Add modifier 26 or TC as appropriate
    Key: d) Add modifier 26 or TC as appropriate
    Explanation: Use appropriate modifier to indicate component provided

86. Complex surgical case includes:
    Laparoscopic appendectomy
    Extensive lysis of adhesions
    Peritoneal drainage
    Choose correct coding:
    a) 44970, 44180
    b) 44970
    c) 44970, 44180-59
    d) 44180, 44970-51
    Key: b) 44970
    Explanation: Lysis and drainage are included in primary procedure when performed at same session.

87. Patient with:
    Sepsis due to MRSA
    Acute respiratory failure
    Acute kidney injury
    Code sequence:

a) A41.02, J96.00, N17.9
b) J96.00, A41.02, N17.9
c) N17.9, A41.02, J96.00
d) A41.02, N17.9, J96.00
Key: a) A41.02, J96.00, N17.9
Explanation: Sepsis coded first, followed by manifestations.

88. Multiple radiology procedures:
CT chest with contrast
CT abdomen with contrast
CT pelvis with contrast
Correct coding:
a) 71260, 74160, 72193
b) 71260, 74177
c) 74177 only
d) 71260, 74178
Key: b) 71260, 74177
Explanation: Combined abd/pelvis CT code with separate chest CT.

89. Preventive visit with:
Annual wellness visit
Problem-oriented service
Immunizations
Code sequence:
a) G0438, 99213-25, 90471
b) G0438 only
c) 99213, 90471
d) G0438, 99213
Key: a) G0438, 99213-25, 90471
Explanation: Separate services with modifier 25 for E/M.

90. Home health certification:
    Initial certification
    Care plan oversight
    Face-to-face visit
    Choose coding:
    a) G0180
    b) G0180, G0181
    c) G0180, 99374
    d) G0180, 99495
    Key: a) G0180
    Explanation: Initial certification includes all components.

91. Anesthesia for:
    Total knee replacement
    Regional block
    Post-op pain management
    Correct coding:
    a) 01402
    b) 01402, 64447
    c) 01402, 64447-59
    d) 01402 only
    Key: a) 01402
    Explanation: Block included in base anesthesia code.

92. Wound care:
    Complex wound assessment
    Negative pressure therapy
    Dressing change
    Code sequence:
    a) 97597, 97605
    b) 97597 only
    c) 97605 only
    d) 97597, 97605, 97597-59

Key: a) 97597, 97605

Explanation: Separate procedures, both billable.

93. Emergency department:
    Critical care (75 minutes)
    Central line placement
    Chest tube insertion
    Code sequence:
    a) 99291, 99292
    b) 99291, 99292, 36556, 32551
    c) 99291, 36556, 32551
    d) 99291 only
    Key: b) 99291, 99292, 36556, 32551
    Explanation: Critical care time plus procedures.

94. Office procedure:
    I&D abscess
    Complex closure
    Local anesthesia
    Code sequence:
    a) 10061, 12031
    b) 10061 only
    c) 10061, 12031-51
    d) 10061, 12031-59
    Key: a) 10061, 12031
    Explanation: Separate procedures at different sites.

95. DME order:
    Hospital bed, semi-electric
    Trapeze bar
    Side rails
    Code sequence:
    a) E0260, E0910, E0305
    b) E0260 only

c) E0260, E0910
d) E0260, E0305
Key: a) E0260, E0910, E0305
Explanation: Each component separately billable.

96. Diabetic patient:
Insulin pump training
Glucose monitor instruction
Nutritional counseling
Code sequence:
a) G0108, G0109, 97802
b) G0108 only
c) G0108, 97802
d) G0108, G0109
Key: a) G0108, G0109, 97802
Explanation: Each service separately billable.

97. Outpatient therapy:
Physical therapy eval
Occupational therapy eval
Speech therapy eval
Code sequence:
a) 97161, 97165, 92521
b) 97161 only
c) Cannot bill same day
d) 97161, 97165
Key: a) 97161, 97165, 92521
Explanation: Different therapy types billable same day.

98. Medication administration:
IV infusion, initial hour
Additional hour
IV push, different drug
Code sequence:

a) 96365, 96366, 96374
b) 96365 only
c) 96365, 96366
d) 96374 only
Key: a) 96365, 96366, 96374
Explanation: All components separately billable.

99. Laboratory tests:
CBC with diff
Comprehensive metabolic panel
Thyroid panel
Code sequence:
a) 85025, 80053, 80076
b) 85025, 80053
c) 80053 only
d) 85025 only
Key: a) 85025, 80053, 80076
Explanation: Each panel separately billable.

100. Mental health:
Psychiatric diagnostic eval
Psychotherapy 45 min
Crisis intervention
Code sequence:
a) 90791, 90834, 90839
b) 90791 only
c) 90834 only
d) 90791, 90834
Key: a) 90791, 90834, 90839
Explanation: Each service separately billable

101. Obstetric care:
Routine prenatal visits
Vaginal delivery

Postpartum care
Code sequence:
a) 59400
b) 59409, 59430
c) 59410
d) 59425, 59409
Key: a) 59400
Explanation: Global OB package includes all components.

102. Orthopedic procedure:
Closed treatment of humeral fracture
Application of cast
X-ray guidance
Code sequence:
a) 24500, 29075
b) 24500 only
c) 24500, 29075, 76000
d) 24500, 76000
Key: a) 24500, 29075
Explanation: Cast application separate, imaging included.

103. Cardiology:
Echocardiogram complete
Doppler flow studies
3D rendering
Code sequence:
a) 93306
b) 93306, 93325
c) 93306, 76376
d) 93306, 93325, 76376
Key: a) 93306
Explanation: Complete echo includes all components.

104. Ophthalmology:

Comprehensive eye exam

Visual field testing

Fundus photography

Code sequence:

a) 92004, 92083, 92250

b) 92004 only

c) 92004, 92083

d) 92083, 92250

Key: a) 92004, 92083, 92250

Explanation: Each diagnostic test separately billable.

105. Dermatology:

Shave removal of lesion

Destruction of warts

Biopsy

Code sequence:

a) 11300, 17110, 11100

b) 11300 only

c) 17110 only

d) 11100 only

Key: a) 11300, 17110, 11100

Explanation: Different procedures at different sites.

106. ENT procedure:

Tonsillectomy

Adenoidectomy

Control of bleeding

Code sequence:

a) 42820

b) 42821

c) 42820, 42870

d) 42821, 42870

Key: b) 42821

Explanation: Combined T&A code, bleeding control included.

107. Neurology:

EEG, extended monitoring

Video recording

Interpretation

Code sequence:

a) 95819

b) 95951

c) 95819, 95957

d) 95951, 95957

Key: b) 95951

Explanation: Extended monitoring includes all components.

108. Pulmonology:

Bronchoscopy with biopsy

BAL

Fluoroscopic guidance

Code sequence:

a) 31623, 31624

b) 31623

c) 31622, 31624

d) 31623, 76000

Key: a) 31623, 31624

Explanation: Separate procedures, guidance included.

109. Gastroenterology:

Upper endoscopy

Biopsy

H. pylori testing

Code sequence:

a) 43239
b) 43235, 43239
c) 43239, 87338
d) 43235 only
Key: a) 43239
Explanation: Endoscopy with biopsy inclusive code.

110. Urology:
Cystoscopy
Bladder biopsy
Stent removal
Code sequence:
a) 52204, 52310
b) 52204
c) 52310
d) 52235
Key: a) 52204, 52310
Explanation: Separate procedures performed.

111. Podiatry:
Bunionectomy
Hammertoe correction
K-wire fixation
Code sequence:
a) 28296, 28285
b) 28296
c) 28285
d) 28296, 28285, 20650
Key: a) 28296, 28285
Explanation: Separate procedures, fixation included.

112. Pain Management:
Epidural injection
Fluoroscopic guidance

Multiple levels
Code sequence:
a) 62311, 77003
b) 62311
c) 62311, 77003, 62319
d) 62319
Key: b) 62311
Explanation: Guidance included in primary procedure.

113. Plastic Surgery:
Scar revision
Complex closure
Adjacent tissue transfer
Code sequence:
a) 13132, 14040
b) 13132
c) 14040
d) 13132, 14040, 15740
Key: a) 13132, 14040
Explanation: Separate reconstructive procedures.

114. Vascular Surgery:
Arterial bypass
Vein harvest
Angiography
Code sequence:
a) 35556
b) 35556, 35572
c) 35556, 75710
d) 35556, 35572, 75710
Key: a) 35556
Explanation: Component procedures included in bypass.

115. Radiation Oncology:
Treatment planning
IMRT delivery
Weekly management
Code sequence:
a) 77301, 77385, 77427
b) 77385
c) 77301, 77385
d) 77427 only
Key: a) 77301, 77385, 77427
Explanation: All components separately billable

116. Multiple surgical procedures same session:
Appendectomy
Hernia repair
Lysis of adhesions
Code with modifiers:
a) 44950, 49505-51, 44005-51
b) 44950, 49505, 44005
c) 44950-51, 49505-51, 44005
d) 44950, 49505-59, 44005-59
Key: a) 44950, 49505-51, 44005-51
Explanation: Primary procedure without modifier, others with -51.

117. Bilateral procedures:
Knee arthroscopy
Meniscectomy
Chondroplasty
Code with modifiers:
a) 29880-50, 29877-50
b) 29880-RT, 29880-LT
c) 29880-50
d) 29880, 29877

Key: a) 29880-50, 29877-50

Explanation: Both procedures performed bilaterally.

118. Return to OR:

Previous appendectomy

Post-op bleeding

Exploratory laparotomy

Code with modifiers:

a) 49002-78

b) 49002

c) 49002-76

d) 49002-79

Key: a) 49002-78

Explanation: Return to OR for related condition.

119. Assistant surgeon:

Total hip replacement

Complex revision

Bone grafting

Code with modifiers:

a) 27134-80

b) 27134-AS

c) 27134-81

d) 27134-82

Key: a) 27134-80

Explanation: Assistant surgeon modifier for MD/DO.

120. Discontinued procedure:

Started laparoscopic

Converted to open

Complications

Code with modifiers:

a) 47562-53

b) 47600

c) 47562-22

d) 47600-53

Key: a) 47562-53

Explanation: Discontinued laparoscopic procedure.

121. Professional component:

Chest x-ray

EKG

Interpretation only

Code with modifiers:

a) 71046-26, 93000-26

b) 71046-26, 93010

c) 71046-TC, 93000-TC

d) 71046, 93000

Key: b) 71046-26, 93010

Explanation: Professional component for x-ray, separate code for EKG reading.

122. E/M with procedure:

Office visit

Minor procedure

Same diagnosis

Code with modifiers:

a) 99213-25, 10060

b) 99213, 10060

c) 99213, 10060-51

d) 10060, 99213

Key: a) 99213-25, 10060

Explanation: E/M with modifier 25 for separate service.

123. Multiple therapy services:

PT evaluation

OT evaluation

Same day
Code with modifiers:
a) 97161, 97165-59
b) 97161, 97165
c) 97161-59, 97165
d) 97161-51, 97165
Key: a) 97161, 97165-59
Explanation: Distinct therapy services require modifier 59.

124. Repeat procedure:
Same day
Same provider
Different session
Code with modifiers:
a) 31622-76
b) 31622-77
c) 31622-59
d) 31622-51
Key: a) 31622-76
Explanation: Repeat procedure same day, same provider.

125. Reduced services:
Planned procedure
Partially completed
Documentation supports
Code with modifiers:
a) 19301-52
b) 19301-53
c) 19301-73
d) 19301-74
Key: a) 19301-52
Explanation: Reduced service, planned reduction.

126. Technical component:
MRI brain
Facility billing
Equipment/tech only
Code with modifiers:
a) 70551-TC
b) 70551-26
c) 70551
d) 70551-51
Key: a) 70551-TC
Explanation: Technical component only.

127. Staged procedures:
Planned stages
Different sessions
Related procedures
Code with modifiers:
a) 15100-58
b) 15100-76
c) 15100-51
d) 15100-59
Key: a) 15100-58
Explanation: Staged procedure modifier.

128. Team surgery:
Complex procedure
Multiple surgeons
Different specialties
Code with modifiers:
a) 22558-66
b) 22558-62
c) 22558-80
d) 22558-82

Key: a) 22558-66

Explanation: Team surgery modifier.

129. Co-surgery:

Two surgeons

Different portions

Same procedure

Code with modifiers:

a) 33510-62

b) 33510-66

c) 33510-80

d) 33510-81

Key: a) 33510-62

Explanation: Co-surgery modifier.

130. Decision for surgery:

Initial encounter

Decision made

Surgery scheduled

Code with modifiers:

a) 99215-57

b) 99215-25

c) 99215-24

d) 99215-53

Key: a) 99215-57

Explanation: Decision for surgery modifier

131. Complex case with multiple diagnoses:

Type 1 diabetes with ketoacidosis

Acute kidney failure

Hypertensive emergency

Correct sequence:

a) E10.10, N17.9, I16.1

b) I16.1, E10.10, N17.9

c) E10.11, I16.1, N17.9
d) N17.9, E10.10, I16.1
Key: a) E10.10, N17.9, I16.1
Explanation: Principal condition with complications first.

132. Trauma case coding:
Multiple rib fractures
Hemothorax
Open wound chest
Sequence with laterality:
a) S22.41XA, S27.1XXA, S21.301A
b) S27.1XXA, S22.41XA, S21.301A
c) S21.301A, S22.41XA, S27.1XXA
d) S22.41XA, S21.301A, S27.1XXA
Key: b) S27.1XXA, S22.41XA, S21.301A
Explanation: Most severe condition first.

133. Oncology treatment:
Chemotherapy administration
Hydration
Anti-emetic administration
Code sequence:
a) 96413, 96360, 96372
b) 96413
c) 96413, 96360
d) 96360, 96413, 96372
Key: a) 96413, 96360, 96372
Explanation: Primary therapy with supportive services.

134. Surgical package:
Pre-op evaluation
Procedure

Post-op care
What's separately billable:
a) Nothing
b) Pre-op only
c) Unrelated E/M
d) Post-op visits
Key: c) Unrelated E/M
Explanation: Only unrelated services during global period.

135. Multiple endoscopic procedures:
EGD with biopsy
Colonoscopy with polyp removal
Same session
Code sequence:
a) 43239, 45385
b) 43235, 45380
c) 43239 only
d) 45385 only
Key: a) 43239, 45385
Explanation: Separate procedures, different anatomical sites.

136. Fracture care:
Closed reduction
Cast application
X-ray guidance
Complete coding:
a) 25605, 29075
b) 25605
c) 25605, 29075, 76000
d) 25605, 76000

Key: b) 25605

Explanation: Global fracture care includes casting and imaging.

137. Telemedicine during PHE:

New patient

Complex visit

Audio-video

Code with modifiers:

a) 99205-95

b) 99205-GT

c) G2012

d) 99205

Key: a) 99205-95

Explanation: New patient visit with telemedicine modifier.

138. Multiple therapy disciplines:

PT evaluation

OT treatment

Speech therapy

Same day coding:

a) 97161, 97530, 92507

b) 97161 only

c) Cannot bill together

d) 97161, 97530

Key: a) 97161, 97530, 92507

Explanation: Different therapy types billable same day.

139. Advanced imaging:

CT chest

CT abdomen

CT pelvis

With contrast:

a) 71260, 74177

b) 71260, 74160, 72193

c) 74178

d) 71260 only

Key: a) 71260, 74177

Explanation: Chest separate, combined abd/pelvis code.

140. Wound care complexity:

Debridement

Negative pressure application

Complex dressing

Code sequence:

a) 97597, 97605

b) 97597

c) 97605

d) 97597, 97605, 97598

Key: a) 97597, 97605

Explanation: Separate procedures for wound care.

141. Labor and delivery:

Admission

Delivery

Postpartum care

Global package:

a) 59400

b) 59409

c) 59410

d) 59425

Key: a) 59400

Explanation: Complete global OB package.

142. Critical care coding:

First 74 minutes

Additional time

Procedures

Code sequence:

a) 99291, 99292

b) 99291

c) 99292

d) 99291, 99292, 36556

Key: a) 99291, 99292

Explanation: Initial and additional time codes.

143. Multiple surgeons:

Complex spine

Different specialties

Same procedure

Modifier usage:

a) -62

b) -66

c) -80

d) -82

Key: a) -62

Explanation: Co-surgery modifier for two surgeons.

144. Emergency department:

Critical condition

Resuscitation

Multiple procedures

Level selection:

a) 99285

b) 99291

c) 99284

d) 99285, 99291

Key: b) 99291

Explanation: Critical care supersedes ED visit.

145. Anesthesia coding:

Base units

Time units
Physical status
Formula components:
a) Base + Time + Modifier
b) Base × Time
c) (Base + Time) × Modifier
d) Base + Time
Key: c) (Base + Time) × Modifier
Explanation: Complete anesthesia formula.

146. Bilateral procedures:
Same procedure
Both sides
One operative session
Correct modifier:
a) -50
b) -RT, -LT
c) -59
d) -51
Key: a) -50
Explanation: Bilateral procedure modifier.

147. Multiple diagnostic tests:
Same session
Different anatomic sites
Technical component
Modifier usage:
a) -TC
b) -26
c) -59
d) -51
Key: a) -TC
Explanation: Technical component modifier.

148. Assistant surgeon:
    Physician assistant
    Complex procedure
    Documentation supports
    Correct modifier:
    a) -AS
    b) -80
    c) -81
    d) -82
    Key: a) -AS
    Explanation: PA assistant surgeon modifier.

149. Preventive services:
    Annual wellness
    Problem-oriented
    Same visit
    Modifier usage:
    a) -25
    b) -57
    c) -59
    d) None needed
    Key: a) -25
    Explanation: Significant separate service modifier.

150. Global surgery:
    Complicated post-op
    Return to OR
    Modifier selection:
    a) -78
    b) -79
    c) -76
    d) -77

Key: a) -78
Explanation: Return to OR related to original procedure

APPENDIX E: COMMON MEDICAL TERMS GLOSSARY

Acute: Sudden onset, severe symptoms, short duration
Adenopathy: Swollen or enlarged lymph nodes
Adhesion: Abnormal band of tissue connecting organs or structures
Anemia: Deficiency of red blood cells or hemoglobin
Angioplasty: Procedure to open blocked blood vessels
Benign: Not cancerous
Biopsy: Removal of tissue for examination
Bradycardia: Abnormally slow heart rate
Bronchitis: Inflammation of bronchial tubes
Carcinoma: Malignant tumor or cancer
Catheter: Tube inserted into body cavity
Chronic: Long-term, recurring condition
Contusion: Bruise
Cyanosis: Bluish discoloration of skin
Debridement: Removal of dead tissue
Dementia: Progressive cognitive decline
Dysphagia: Difficulty swallowing
Dysplasia: Abnormal cell growth
Edema: Swelling caused by fluid retention
Embolism: Blockage in blood vessel
Encephalitis: Brain inflammation
Erythema: Redness of skin
Fibrillation: Irregular heartbeat
Fistula: Abnormal connection between organs
Fracture: Broken bone
Gangrene: Death of body tissue
Gastritis: Stomach lining inflammation
Graft: Transplanted tissue
Hematoma: Blood collection outside vessels
Hemoptysis: Coughing up blood
Hypertension: High blood pressure

Hypoxia: Oxygen deficiency
Infarction: Tissue death from lack of blood
Inflammation: Tissue response to injury
Ischemia: Reduced blood supply
Lesion: Abnormal tissue change
Lymphadenitis: Lymph node inflammation
Malignant: Cancerous
Metastasis: Spread of cancer
Myalgia: Muscle pain
Necrosis: Cell/tissue death
Neoplasm: New abnormal growth
Neuropathy: Nerve disease
Obstruction: Blockage
Osteoporosis: Bone density loss
Osteomyelitis: Bone infection
Pallor: Paleness
Paralysis: Loss of muscle function
Perforation: Hole through tissue
Pneumonia: Lung inflammation
Remission: Disease symptom reduction
Rupture: Tear or break in tissue
Sepsis: Systemic infection
Stenosis: Narrowing
Syndrome: Group of related symptoms
Thrombosis: Blood clot formation
Tumor: Abnormal mass
Ulcer: Open sore
Uremia: Kidney failure condition
Varicose: Enlarged, twisted veins
Vertigo: Dizziness
Wheal: Raised, itchy area of skin
Wheeze: High-pitched breathing sound
White Matter: Inner part of brain/spinal cord containing nerve fibers
Xanthelasma: Yellow patches around eyelids

Xerosis: Abnormal dryness, especially of skin
Xerostomia: Dry mouth condition
Yellow Fever: Viral infection causing jaundice
Yeast Infection: Fungal infection
Yield Point: Point at which tissue begins to deform permanently
Zoonosis: Disease transmitted from animals to humans
Zoster: Shingles (Herpes zoster)
Zygomatic: Relating to the cheekbone
Zygote: Fertilized egg cell

APPENDIX F: ABBREVIATIONS LIST

a.c. (ante cibum) - before meals
ABG - Arterial Blood Gas
ADL - Activities of Daily Living
AMA - Against Medical Advice
AP - Anterior/Posterior
b.i.d. (bis in die) - twice a day
BMI - Body Mass Index
BP - Blood Pressure
BUN - Blood Urea Nitrogen
C&S - Culture and Sensitivity
CAD - Coronary Artery Disease
CBC - Complete Blood Count
CHF - Congestive Heart Failure
COPD - Chronic Obstructive Pulmonary Disease
CT - Computed Tomography
CVA - Cerebrovascular Accident
D&C - Dilation and Curettage
DM - Diabetes Mellitus
DNR - Do Not Resuscitate
DOA - Dead On Arrival
DVT - Deep Vein Thrombosis
ECG/EKG - Electrocardiogram
ED - Emergency Department
ENT - Ear, Nose, and Throat
ESR - Erythrocyte Sedimentation Rate
FB - Foreign Body
FH - Family History
FUO - Fever of Unknown Origin
GI - Gastrointestinal
GSW - Gunshot Wound
GTT - Glucose Tolerance Test
H&P - History and Physical
Hb/Hgb - Hemoglobin
HTN - Hypertension

Hx - History
I&D - Incision and Drainage
I&O - Intake and Output
ICU - Intensive Care Unit
IM - Intramuscular
IV - Intravenous
L&D - Labor and Delivery
LAT - Left Anterior Thorax
LMP - Last Menstrual Period
LOC - Loss of Consciousness
MI - Myocardial Infarction
MRI - Magnetic Resonance Imaging
MVA - Motor Vehicle Accident
N&V - Nausea and Vomiting
NPO - Nothing by Mouth
NSAID - Non-Steroidal Anti-Inflammatory Drug
OB/GYN - Obstetrics/Gynecology
OOB - Out of Bed
OR - Operating Room
p.c. - after meals
p.o. - by mouth
P.R.N. - as needed
PERLA - Pupils Equal, React to Light and Accommodation
PT - Physical Therapy
q.d. - every day
q.h. - every hour
q.i.d. - four times a day
R/O - Rule Out
RBC - Red Blood Cell
ROS - Review of Systems
Rx - Prescription
SOB - Shortness of Breath
S/P - Status Post
STAT - Immediately

Sx - Symptoms
T&A - Tonsillectomy and Adenoidectomy
TIA - Transient Ischemic Attack
TPR - Temperature, Pulse, Respiration
URI - Upper Respiratory Infection
UTI - Urinary Tract Infection
VS - Vital Signs
VSD - Ventricular Septal Defect
WBC - White Blood Cell
WNL - Within Normal Limits
W/O - Without
XR - X-Ray

APPENDIX G: QUICK REFERENCE GUIDELINES

General Coding Guidelines

- Review complete medical record before coding
- Code to highest level of specificity
- Default to unspecified code only when no other information is available
- Follow Excludes1 and Excludes2 notes carefully
- Check for combination codes before assigning separate codes

Sequencing Rules

- Code principal diagnosis first
- Code conditions that affect treatment
- Follow "code first" and "use additional code" instructions
- Sequence acute conditions before chronic
- Code complications after the condition

Documentation Requirements

- Confirm physician documentation before coding
- Never code from diagnostic test results alone
- Documentation must support medical necessity
- Query provider for clarification when needed
- Document any missing or conflicting information

Chapter-Specific Guidelines

a) Neoplasms

- Code site first
- Use additional code for functional activity
- Sequence primary malignancy first when present

b) Injuries

- Code site and type of injury

- Include external cause codes
- Code initial vs. subsequent encounter
- Document left, right, or bilateral when applicable

c) Pregnancy

- Always use Chapter 15 codes first
- Document trimester
- Include outcome of delivery when applicable

Common ICD-10 Sections

- A00-B99: Infectious/parasitic diseases
- C00-D49: Neoplasms
- I00-I99: Circulatory system
- J00-J99: Respiratory system
- K00-K95: Digestive system
- M00-M99: Musculoskeletal system
- S00-T88: Injury, poisoning, external causes

APPENDIX H: IMPORTANT MODIFIERS

Evaluation & Management Modifiers

- 24: Unrelated E/M service during postoperative period
- 25: Significant, separately identifiable E/M service
- 57: Decision for surgery

Anatomical Modifiers

- LT: Left side
- RT: Right side
- 50: Bilateral procedure
- E1-E4: Eyelids
- FA-F9: Fingers
- TA-T9: Toes

Service/Procedure Modifiers

- 22: Increased procedural services
- 26: Professional component
- 51: Multiple procedures
- 52: Reduced services
- 53: Discontinued procedure
- 58: Staged/related procedure
- 59: Distinct procedural service
- 76: Repeat procedure by same physician
- 77: Repeat procedure by another physician
- 78: Return to OR for related procedure
- 79: Unrelated procedure during postoperative period

Payment Modifiers

- AS: Assistant surgeon
- 62: Co-surgeon
- 80: Assistant surgeon
- 81: Minimum assistant surgeon

- 82: Assistant surgeon (when qualified resident unavailable)

Place of Service Modifiers

- 23: Emergency department
- 24: Ambulatory surgical center
- 26: Military treatment facility
- 31: Skilled nursing facility
- 32: Nursing facility

Special Circumstances Modifiers

- AI: Principal physician
- CC: Procedure code change
- GC: Teaching physician present
- GE: Services performed by resident
- QW: CLIA waived test

Informational Modifiers

- 90: Reference laboratory
- 91: Repeat clinical diagnostic laboratory test
- 92: Alternative laboratory platform testing
- 99: Multiple modifiers

APPENDIX I: CPC EXAM RESOURCES

Exam Overview

- 5 hours and 40 minutes duration
- 150 multiple-choice questions
- 70% passing score required (105 correct answers)
- Open book examination
- No electronic devices allowed

Essential Study Materials

a) Required Resources

- Current year ICD-10-CM coding manual
- Current year CPT coding manual
- Current year HCPCS Level II manual

b) Recommended Study Guides

- Official CPC Study Guide
- Practice exam bundles
- Medical terminology workbooks
- Anatomy and physiology review materials

Exam Content Distribution

- Medical Terminology: 11%
- Anatomy and Physiology: 11%
- ICD-10-CM Guidelines: 9%
- CPT Coding: 47%
- HCPCS Level II: 5%
- Compliance and Regulatory: 10%
- E/M Services: 7%

Key Study Areas

a) CPT Sections

- Evaluation and Management
- Anesthesia
- Surgery

- Radiology
- Pathology/Laboratory
- Medicine

b) Anatomy Systems

- Integumentary
- Musculoskeletal
- Respiratory
- Cardiovascular
- Digestive
- Urinary
- Reproductive
- Endocrine
- Nervous System

Test-Taking Strategies

a) Time Management

- Read questions carefully
- Budget approximately 2 minutes per question
- Mark difficult questions for review
- Complete easier questions first
- Leave time for review

b) Process of Elimination

- Eliminate obviously incorrect answers
- Look for key words in questions
- Pay attention to code descriptors
- Check guidelines carefully
- Verify correct modifiers

Practice Tips

- Complete at least 3 full practice exams
- Time yourself during practice
- Review missed questions thoroughly
- Focus on weak areas
- Study guidelines and conventions

- Practice using index and tabular sections

Exam Day Preparation

a) What to Bring

- Current coding manuals
- Pencils and eraser
- Watch for time management
- Clear drinking water
- Light snack

b) Manual Organization

- Tab important sections
- Highlight frequently used codes
- Mark important guidelines
- Create quick reference notes
- Index frequently used modifiers

Post-Exam Resources

- CPC exam retake policy
- Continuing education requirements
- AAPC membership benefits
- Local chapter meetings
- Certification maintenance

Common Exam Topics

- Bundle vs. Unbundle procedures
- Correct modifier usage
- Multiple procedure coding
- Global surgical package
- Medical necessity documentation
- Compliance regulations
- Coverage determinations
- Medical terminology roots
- Anatomical positions
- Surgical approaches

Online Resources

- AAPC website practice questions
- Coding webinars
- Discussion forums
- Study groups
- Virtual practice exams

ANSWERS TO THE MCQS

Chapter 1

1. b
2. c
3. d
4. c
5. c
6. c
7. c
8. c
9. b
10. b
11. c
12. c
13. b
14. c
15. c
16. b
17. c
18. c
19. b
20. b
21. c
22. c
23. b
24. c
25. c

Chapter 2

1. b
2. b
3. c
4. b
5. b
6. c
7. c
8. c
9. b
10. b
11. b
12. b
13. c
14. b
15. b
16. b
17. b
18. c
19. b
20. a
21. b
22. b
23. b
24. c
25. b

Chapter 3

1. b
2. d
3. c
4. a
5. b
6. b
7. c
8. b
9. c
10. b
11. b
12. b
13. b
14. b
15. c
16. c
17. b
18. c
19. b
20. b
21. b
22. b
23. c
24. b
25. a

Chapter 4

1. b
2. c
3. b
4. c
5. c
6. c
7. c
8. b
9. b
10. c
11. c
12. c
13. b
14. c
15. c
16. b
17. c
18. b
19. c
20. b
21. b
22. c
23. c

24. c
25. c

Chapter 5

1. b
2. c
3. b
4. c
5. b
6. b
7. b
8. c
9. b
10. c
11. b
12. a
13. b
14. c
15. b
16. c
17. b
18. b
19. b
20. a
21. c
22. c
23. a
24. b
25. c

Chapter 6

1. b
2. b
3. c
4. a
5. c
6. b
7. d
8. a
9. b
10. b
11. b
12. a
13. b
14. c
15. b
16. b
17. a
18. c
19. c
20. b
21. a
22. c
23. a
24. b
25. d

Chapter 7

1. b
2. b
3. a
4. c
5. c
6. b
7. b
8. c
9. a
10. c
11. b
12. a
13. c
14. d
15. c
16. b
17. b
18. c
19. b
20. c
21. d
22. b
23. d
24. b
25. c

Chapter 8

1. b
2. b
3. b
4. c
5. c
6. d
7. b
8. b
9. b
10. b
11. b
12. c
13. c
14. c
15. d
16. c
17. b
18. d
19. b
20. b
21. b
22. c

23. a
24. d
25. a

Chapter 9

1. b
2. b
3. b
4. c
5. c
6. c
7. b
8. a
9. d
10. c
11. b
12. b
13. b
14. c
15. d
16. b
17. b
18. b
19. c
20. b
21. c
22. d
23. b
24. b
25. c

Chapter 10

1. b
2. b
3. b
4. b
5. b
6. d
7. c
8. d
9. b
10. a
11. c
12. c
13. c
14. c
15. c
16. c
17. c
18. b
19. c
20. b
21. c
22. c
23. c
24. b
25. c

Chapter 11

1. b
2. b
3. b
4. c
5. b
6. c
7. a
8. c
9. c
10. b
11. b
12. d
13. a
14. b
15. c
16. c
17. b
18. b
19. c
20. c
21. a
22. b
23. d
24. c
25. c

Chapter 12

1. c)
2. b)
3. c)
4. c)
5. b)
6. c)
7. a)
8. b)
9. c)
10. c)
11. c)
12. c)
13. b)
14. c)
15. b)
16. b)
17. c)
18. b)
19. c)
20. c)
21. c)
22. c)
23. c)
24. c)
25. b)

ABOUT THE EDITORS

Dr. SOWJANYA GURUGUBELLI

Dr. Sowjanya Gurugubelli holds a B. Pharmacy, M.Tech in Biotechnology (JNTU Hyderabad), and Ph.D in Pharmaceutical Sciences (Andhra University). An Associate Professor at Aditya Pharmacy College with over 10 years of teaching experience, she received a National Award at APTICON-2022. Dr. Sowjanya has participated in DST-funded STUTI-21, published 7 research articles, presented at various conferences, and is a reviewer for two journals. She is a lifetime member of two professional bodies.

Mrs. VINNY THERISSA MANGAM

Mrs. Vinny Therissa Mangam is an Assistant Professor working at Aditya College of Pharmacy, Aditya University with over 4 years of experience in teaching, analytical method development and validation. She published 8 research papers and lifetime member of APT and IPGA. Her expertise lies in optimizing techniques, comparing methods, and transferring procedures to enable enhanced standards in pharmaceutical analysis.

Mr. PRAKASH NATHANIEL KUMAR SARELLA

Mr. Prakash Nathaniel Kumar Sarella is working as an Associate Professor at Aditya College of Pharmacy, Aditya University with over 8 years of experience in teaching and research. His expertise includes nanomedicine, liposomes, polymer therapeutics, antibody-drug conjugates, and microneedle technologies, and other innovative drug delivery solutions. He published over 40 research papers and life member of APTI and IPGA.

Mr. GOURAB SAHA

Mr. Gourab Saha serves as an Assistant Professor in the Department of Pharmaceutics at the College of Pharmaceutical Sciences, Berhampur, where he also completed his B.Pharm and M.Pharm degrees. With teaching experience since 2013, he has participated in multiple national and international conferences in pharmaceutical sciences.

Dr. SYED AFZAL UDDIN BIYABANI

Dr. Syed Afzal Uddin Biyabani, a research scholar at Rajiv Gandhi University of Health Sciences in Bangalore, is an expert in pharmacy and health sciences. He has authored three key books: 'Foundation of Pharmacy and Health Sciences,' 'Emergency Toxicology,' and 'Pharmacotherapeutics-3 for PharmD 4th Year.' His work focuses on advancing pharmaceutical education and toxicology management.

www.ingramcontent.com/pod-product-compliance
Lightning Source LLC
Chambersburg PA
CBHW062132160726
48282CB00027B/800
9788197973192